SEXUAL EVOLUTION

SEXUAL EVOLUTION
Sexual Evolution

Rhonda Levand

CELESTIAL ARTS
Berkeley, California

CELESTIAL ARTS
P.O. Box 7327
Berkeley, California 94707

Cover design by Ken Scott
Cover art by Helena Gibson
Composition by The Recorder Typesetting Network

Library of Congress Cataloging-in-Publication Data

Levand, Rhonda
Sexual evolution / Rhonda Levand.
p. cm.
Includes bibliographical references.
ISBN 0-89087-626-6
1. Sex (Psychology)—Case studies. 2. Psychosexual development—Case studies. 3. Childbirth—Psychological aspects—Case studies. 4. Conception—Psychological aspects—Case studies. 5. Interpersonal relations—Case studies. 6. Sex therapy—Case studies. I. Title.
BF692.L524 1991
155.3—dc20 90-2338
CIP

First Printing 1991

0 9 8 7 6 5 4 3 2 1
95 94 93 92 91

Manufactured in the United States of America

DEDICATION

SEXUAL EVOLUTION means lightening up on sex, and having more fun, bliss, excitement, energy and aliveness in our lives. Being enlightened means lightening up on our thoughts. Since our thoughts create our experience, sexual evolution is the process of becoming enlightened about our thoughts, about sex and about our sexuality.

We all take sex too seriously. It often becomes a hard, tremendous issue in people's lives. The purpose of this book is to help us all lighten up on sex and to see why and where we decided it was difficult, hard and a struggle.

This book is dedicated to all those people who have helped me to lighten up on sex and my life, especially my parents Jack and Gloria Levand, Sondra Ray, Babaji, Bob and Mallie Mandel, my children Raynbow and Jarrett Schleyer, and Jeffrey Baker, my enlightened sexual partner.

ACKNOWLEDGEMENTS

THE AUTHOR acknowledges and is grateful to: Sondra Ray for her continued support in the creation and completion of this book; Bob Mandel for his practical and creative input and his inspiration for the title *Sexual Evolution*; Mallie Mandel for proofreading; Nanci DeLucrezia for editing the first draft; Kathy Arnos for her support and many hours of work putting the first draft in the computer; Lane Watts for his additional computer work; Penelope Court for her organizational skills and computer work needed for the completion of this book.

The author also acknowledges and thanks all the people from around the world who contributed their sexual histories and stories to make this book a reality.

CONTENTS

PREFACE

WHEN I WAS a sex therapist in California back in the 1970s, the market was already flooded with sex books. My publishers were hesitant to take a chance on publishing another sex book. But I knew that my manuscript, *I Deserve Love*, was different and important. I convinced my publishers that what we needed out there were enlightened sex books, books that produced results by getting to the actual CAUSE of sex problems. At the time I was doing innovative work in the use of affirmations to heal sexual issues . . . and it was effective. My publishers took a chance on me and the book. Now it is one of the best sellers in that publishing house.

After I became a rebirther, I realized that I had only scratched the surface in this field. As I began to research the effects of one's birth trauma on relationships, I was absolutely startled at the profound information we rebirthers began learning on this subject. I began to write more books and put this information in seminars, especially the Loving Relationships Training. However, I suddenly became so busy that I was unable to do the specific research necessary in the area of sexuality.

When I saw Rhonda's natural interest in the subject and enthusiasm for carrying out her work, I new she had the energy and makeup for this work. So I asked her to write a book and she eagerly took on the project. I really want to acknowledge her contribution. I am sure you as a reader will benefit greatly from her research. I know for a fact that you will receive much benefit from all her energy which pours through from behind the words. Her joy and enthusiasm for life contributes to everyone, and I would certainly recommend that you attend any of her seminars that are given in your area.

Naturally we all welcome any information that you can add to this research, so please feel free to let us know any more insights you have in regards to the subject of how conception, birth and infancy effect your sex life. Rebirthing is only in its second decade, and we are still learning and will continue to be open to expanding this information.

After being a rebirther for fourteen years I can vouch for the fact that your birth has more power over you than almost anything you can talk about. But until you get rebirthed, you might not be aware of that at all, because it seems like that is just the way life is. . . .

At first, we rebirthers were quite amazed at how rebirthing can improve your sex life. It was one of the great side benefits that we did not expect. Not only can rebirthing improve your sex life, which you may feel is working fairly well, but it certainly can correct any sexual issues that trouble you. The bottom line of any sexual issue is to find out the cause of the problem. Often this cause is so much deeper than we realize. It may be surprising at first to hear that sexual issues probably go all the way back to conception, pregnancy and birth. But if you stop and think about it a few minutes it will rapidly make sense to you.

Rhonda's years of experience as a gifted rebirther and LRT Trainer qualify her as the perfect person to put this information together. We in the LRT community are all very grateful to her.

—Sondra Ray

INTRODUCTION

ONE'S SEXUALITY IS usually kept private and undiscussed. The purpose of sharing my sexual history and the sexual histories of persons who have taken sexuality weekends is to enhance, support and stimulate people reading this book to discover insights into their own sexuality.

My sexual exploits and history are not necessarily something I am proud of, or can easily share with the whole world. I have learned about myself and others by looking deeply into what I have done sexually in my past. My willingness to tell the truth about my sexual history has allowed me to have more pleasure and bliss in my intimate relationships.

My sexuality was a problem for me. Loving, approving and accepting myself as a beautiful, sexy and lovable woman was a major step toward healing my sexual issues.

Over the past three years I have led dozens of trainings: Loving Relationships Trainings, sexuality weekends and rebirthing trainings. I have shared myself and my stories. This is the easiest way I found to teach what I need to learn, master and grow myself, and support others in their personal growth process. I have always been acknowledged by participants of the trainings I have led for how much they related to my stories and how these stories helped them to look deeper at a part of themselves.

The following is a letter I received from a student in London after a Loving Relationships Training I led there with Fredric Lehrman.

> Dear Rhonda and Fred,
>
> Thank you very, very much for the LRT. During the training not a lot seemed to be happening for me. But now afterwards I feel that "something" has happened anyway!

> I want especially to thank you, Rhonda, for sharing the part about wanting to be a boy. I find that my whole left side is in pain and my left eye has been inflamed right into the cornea for two years and more!
>
> My mother had a boy miscarriage just before I was conceived (my boy body). They also called me little Jimmy the football player in the womb! I was going to share this, but the moment passed. My eye and my body were what brought me to the LRT.
>
> I'm now doing affirmations on my femaleness from the book *You Can Heal Your Life*. Do you have any other suggestions for me? (I have also had chronic weight loss these past years.)
>
> Lovingly, Susan

Susan realized in the LRT how she was blocking her feminine energy. This blocking was expressed through the problems she had on the left side of her body. The left side represents the feminine side of each of us. My sharing triggered her recognition of how she had rejected her feminine self because of a similar issue. Through this recognition she was able to get to the cause of her problems with her left eye and left side. Once she recognized the cause of the problem she could embrace her feminine self and heal her body.

I decided to write a book on sexuality to learn more about myself, and to support others in healing an aspect of their lives that is often suppressed and denied—our sexual aliveness and energy. This book has been a three-year process from the time I decided to write it to the time it got to the publisher.

Over the past three years I have interviewed people about their sexuality. People in my sexuality weekends and longer rebirthing trainings have done written assignments about their sexuality which are included in this book. Each one of us is unique and different, and at the same time we share similarities and can relate to each other on a very deep level. The purpose of including a wide range of sexual histories and stories is to show that we are all different and at the same time a part of each other. As I read over other people's histories I discovered how much we all do have in common with each other. I related to part of the story of each person who contributed to this book.

Often we feel that we are alone, separate, unique, and no one would understand what we are going through, especially about our sexuality. The truth is that the more people share in trainings about themselves sexually, the better and more connected everyone feels. People see that they no longer have to feel guilty, different or strange about what is going on with them sexually.

The purpose of this book is to show you how normal, sane and sexually healthy you really are. You are not alone. We all have things going on that we would like to change, heal and make better in our lives.

I invite and challenge you to look at yourself through my eyes as well as through the eyes of all the people contributing their sexual histories to this book.

If you gain one good insight about yourself through reading this book of sexual histories, and learn how to change in a positive direction toward more sexual bliss and pleasure, the effort of reading this book has been worth it.

I would like to acknowledge all the people from all over the world—Australia, New Zealand, Sweden, England, France, Germany, California, Florida, Washington state, Alaska, and Georgia—who have contributed their sexual histories to this book for the purpose of healing themselves and you.

Once I decided to write this book it evolved easily. I would finish one chapter and the idea for the next chapter would come to me and flow onto the paper. I just looked back on my own life and related each aspect of my development to my sexuality.

This made sense to me since I had a Masters Degree in the Psychology of Early Childhood. This book is a study of how our early childhoods affect us in our lives as adults. Of course, after I became a rebirther, I also discovered the importance of conception, the intro-uterine period, and birth in our adult lives, and specifically in our sex lives.

In the Loving Relationships Training we say that what you focus on expands. If you focus on having a more blissful, orgasmic, pleasurable sex life, that will be the outcome for you of reading this book.

The premise of this book is that we are the creators of our lives. We choose our sex, our parents, our environment, and whether or not we will be happy, prosperous and successful. We create our sexual histories, which start at the moment we are conceived. Our sexual attitudes and happenings are affected by what happened to us at conception, in the womb, at birth, in infancy and early childhood. We are making very sophisticated decisions about our sexuality before we have any conscious memories.

Our lives are like a movie. The film we put into the projector to create our own personal movie consists of all the unconscious decisions we made at conception, in the womb, at birth, and during infancy and early childhood. Our lives keep playing the same movie over and over again because our mind is projecting the past onto the screen of the present. Our sex lives are the result of every bit of information we have gathered from conception to the present.

In order to have enlightened, cosmic, joyous sex, we must be willing to take responsibility for creating it that way. I went from being a non-orgasmic woman who did not accept fully being a woman, to being a multiple-orgasmic woman totally in love with my femininity and sexuality. I didn't get there by taking classes on sexual technique. I got there by learning how to master creative thought. In other words, since I created being non-orgasmic, I could also create being multi-orgasmic. I did this by totally accepting responsibility for my life and seeing that I choose it every step of the way. So let's start right at the beginning and look at how that works.

CHAPTER 1

Conception

Our First Encounter with Sex

I AM SURE most of you think you don't remember your conception. But just think about it for a minute. All the information about your conception is available to you as soon as you realize it is and ask for it. Conception was our first encounter with sex.

Our parents were making love and out of their sexual union we were created. If their sexual experience was enlightened, loving, innocent, conscious and totally satisfying, what decision would we have made about sex—since we were totally conscious beings even then? We would understand that sex was innocent, enlightening, loving, conscious and totally satisfying. Unfortunately most of us were not conceived in this way. Let's look at some different kinds of conceptions.

What would your decision be about sex if your mother was raped, hurt or made love to in a very unconscious way? You would have a totally different concept of sex. You could even create being sexually abused or raped in your own life.

Some other issues that are important to look at around conception are whether you were planned or wanted, whether you were a financial burden, and whether you were illegitimate or an accident. Did your parents want a boy when you were a girl, or vice versa? All of the circumstances and thoughts your parents had at your conception are important to know in understanding what makes you click sexually.

My parents wanted a boy, so that although I was planned, I always had confusion around being a woman. I made the decision that in order to please my parents, I had to be the opposite of what I was—a boy. I tried being a tomboy. My parents' thought of wanting a boy affected how I looked at my sexuality. Since I didn't think I was supposed to be a woman, I found it difficult to surrender and receive pleasure with a man. I acted this out in many ways. I would try to be the giver and dominate my sexual partner, pleasing the man, but never myself. I would go through the motions but not really be there to give or receive. I experimented sexually with many men to prove that I was wanted as a woman. None of these ways were satisfying or fulfilling.

In order to have joyous, pleasurable sex, women must accept their femininity. They both receive and give in the sexual act. Giving and receiving are the same, so whatever we give, we receive. Being feminine is being able to receive. In order to have orgasmic sex, a woman has to open up to her femininity and be willing to surrender and trust her partner completely. This means giving up control; being willing to be out of control. If she is unconsciously trying to be a man, this can't happen.

Many women can have clitoral orgasms, but not vaginal orgasms. I believe this is because the clitoris is like a little penis, and represents the male part of a woman's sexual equipment—so women who have not completely accepted their femininity can't experience orgasms at all, or experience only clitorial orgasms.

However, when we surrender to our womanhood and acknowledge that we chose to be women, we learn to receive men and trust them completely sexually. We can then experience orgasms that shoot through our whole bodies.

Since I thought I was supposed to be a boy, I also kept my breasts from being full and sexually sensitive. The more I accepted the fact that I chose to be a woman—the more sensitive and fuller my breasts became. I became able to have orgasms by just having my breasts touched.

Breasts represent the fullness and ripeness of womanhood and are one of our sexiest attributes. When we don't acknowledge our womanhood, we inhibit our sensitivity in this very erotic part of our bodies. It's important to love every part of our bodies in order to experience the full pleasure and joy sex can bring.

If a man's parents wanted a girl, he could have difficulty in fully accepting his masculinity. Instead of wanting to be the giver he could be more passive, and want to receive all the time. He might have a fear of realizing the male sexual being that he is. He may have the thought that he hurt his parents by being a man, and hold back his power and sexuality. He may be only sexually satisfied if his partner is the aggressor in the sexual encounter, and find he has no drive, or very little.

In the process of letting go of my confusion about my sexuality, I attracted a lot of gay men into my life. I even felt I was in love with a bisexual man.

He was reflecting my inner uncertainty about whether I wanted to be a man or a woman. He had a difficult choice to make between me and his male lover. This outside confusion showed me exactly what was going on inside of me—my sexual identity confusion.

My experience with homosexual men is that there is a lot of sexual confusion. I could relate to them because I had the same confusion. That is why I attracted so many homosexuals into my life—to mirror my own confusion. Many of these men shared that their parents wanted girls. They often had the thought that they hurt women, and felt guilty about it. They decided they had to stay away from women so they wouldn't hurt them and be guilty.

I love to be around gay men because they are sensitive, creative, intuitive and spiritual. They have really cultivated their feminine side. I do feel homosexuality starts at conception—that one comes into life choosing to be homosexual. The important thing to remember if you are gay is that you chose it, just as the rest of us chose heterosexuality. So you have the choice at anytime to stay homosexual or to choose heterosexuality. Once you realize that you can choose, you can experience your innocence completely, and really decide what you want sexually.

If a person's conception happened during a one night stand, out of wedlock, or was an accident, the decision made about sex would be very different from the decision made in a conception rooted in deep love and commitment. The sex lives of these people could be a sucession of one night stands or affairs, or their relationships could have a lack of commitment. The decisions made could create unsatisfying sexual encounters and the thought that you are not really wanted for anything but sex. The encounter just happened by accident. This kind of decision would make it difficult to trust, or to surrender completely to a partner sexually. The fear would be that it could end as quickly as it began.

I have known people who had an accidental or illegitimate conception who recreate this circumstance and have an illegitimate child of their own. The thought is that if I have sex I will create an illegitimate child because that was how I was created. Often these people will stay away from the pleasure of sex to avoid the fear of pregnancy.

Sometimes conception is an accident, the parents are not ready, and the child is a financial burden. The decision here could be that since I started out as a financial burden, I can't help becoming a financial burden to every person I am sexual with. Often sex and money are closely tied together. Many times people get involved sexually with someone so they can be taken care of financially.

Often parents choose to conceive a child to save a troubled marriage, and then the marriage fails anyway. Their child may feel that having sex is a way to keep a relationship together, which is a set-up for failure. When a person has the thought that "I was brought into this world to save my parents' marriage, I came and did everything right and it didn't work," the person could do everything right to save their adult relationship sexually and still lose out.

One of the ways to heal these conception thoughts is to accept that you chose the sex that you are and all the circumstances of your conception. There are several affirmations that change the old conception thoughts. An affirmation is a positive thought that we plant in our consciousness in order to release our old decisions. The more we get in touch with the old decisions we made about our sexuality, the more we become empowered as the men and women we are.

The reason I chose to be a woman, when my parents wanted a boy, was because I knew deep down that women would be the teachers in the Age of Enlightenment. We have just shifted from the male-dominated Age of Pisces or Age of Reason, to the intuitive, creative, emotional and spiritual Age of Enlightenment, the Golden Age. I realize I chose to be a woman when the age shifted. I understood my purpose and mission as a woman. I saw how valuable I was as a woman. I also had already learned a lot about my masculine side by trying to be my father's son. So now I am coming into balance by enhancing my feminine side.

Here are some of the affirmations I used to make the shift to come into more balance. Sex becomes more enlightened and pleasurable when we are internally in balance with our feminine and masculine sides.

Affirmations for Conception Trauma

1. I now see that I chose to be a man (or woman).
2. I accept, want, and love myself completely as a woman (or man).
3. I chose my sexuality—I celebrate my femininity (or masculinity).
4. Because I want myself as a man (or woman), I can have what I want sexually.
5. I am what I want and what my partner wants sexually.
6. Since I chose to be here I can have what I want sexually.
7. I love both my feminine and masculine sides.
8. I now acknowledge my femininity and masculinity.
9. My sexuality is innocent.

10. I can have sex the way I choose it.

11. The conception of my sexuality is perfect.

Choose the affirmations you want. Work with one or two at the same time. Write each affirmation twenty times a day for one week using a response column. You know that you have integrated your affirmation when you have no more negative responses in the response column. Then you can have the results in your life you want, for you will no longer have anger about your sexuality and you can enjoy sex more.

Example of an Affirmation with a Response Column

AFFIRMATION	RESPONSE
1. I completely accept, love and want myself as a woman.	1. But my parents wanted a boy.
2. I completely accept, love and want myself as a woman.	2. Men are more powerful.
3. I completely accept, love and want myself as a woman.	3. Men get what they want; women don't.
4. I completely accept, love and want myself as a woman.	4. Being a woman is OK.
5. I completely accept, love and want myself as a woman.	5. It's great!

The Conception and Birth of My Relationship with Jeffrey

In August of 1986, Jeff and I went to New York to attend a Couple's Ten-Day Intensive Seminar with Bob and Mallie Mandel (two trainers with the Loving Relationships Training). At that time we had been in a relationship for about five months. We had some fear about going to the couple's seminar, because things were so good we didn't want to ruin it or make it hard. We were a little afraid to stir things up and maybe find out our relationship wasn't as perfect as we thought it was.

The reality was that the couple's seminar strengthened our relationship, and gave us many tools for enhancing our already close, intimate bond. At the intensive, we got lots of recognition for how wonderful our relationship really was. During it, we focused on all the good in our relationship, and since what you focus on expands, after that ten days we felt even more bonded and safer with each other.

The main thing I learned in the seminar about our relationship and myself was about my conception trauma. One day in class we were asked to share about the conception of our relationship with the group. I was really excited about this, but Jeff was very reluctant to share. The more couples shared about the wonderful, magical conceptions of their relationships, the more reluctant Jeff became about sharing. He was hoping we wouldn't have to do this because the end of class was approaching. I found myself getting really angry at him. My body felt terrible and I started pushing him away. I felt if the conception of the relationship wasn't good enough, maybe the whole relationship wasn't good enough.

After class we rode out to New Jersey with another couple to spend the night at their house. We were going to rebirth each other that evening. I was sitting in the back seat just seething—smoke was almost coming out of me. The three of them were talking. Jeff was practically afraid to look at me. At one point he asked if I was alright. I was so angry I almost bit his head off. I could not verbalize what was going on with me because I was so hurt and angry. I wasn't in touch with what was going on yet.

After I got through these feelings I started to understand that I was re-experiencing my actual conception. I knew that when my parents conceived me, their intention was to have a son. (I guess I had a different idea because I chose to be a girl.) I knew this intellectually, but the experience at the couple's seminar allowed me to re-experience my disappointment in not pleasing them and not being what they wanted. I was enthusiastic about being their child and being a girl, but they were not so excited about me initially.

Jeff brought those feelings up for me. What he felt was that our conception was not good enough to share because it was not magical like many of the conception stories. Being an actor Jeff wanted something dramatic, magical or exciting to act out in front of the group. He thought our conception was no big deal and would probably be a disappointment.

We were off balance. I was excited and he wasn't about the conception of our relationship, just as I had been excited about my parents, but they hadn't been too excited about me.

Anyway, we were driving to New Jersey, and all of a sudden I really felt sad, and started to cry as we went through the Holland Tunnel. I realized I was in the birth canal, and I was sad and afraid to come out because I knew my parents wanted a boy. Five minutes after we were out of the tunnel, I felt better. Then I realized why I had felt so upset and terrible about what happened in the conception process. Momentarily my parents had been disappointed that I was a girl, but then instantly they had loved me and been happy. I was healthy. They were thrilled with me.

I, however, unconsciously made the decision that I wasn't what they wanted at the beginning, but after they knew me they really loved me. I have re-created this over and over again in relationships. Men at first are not attracted to me sexually or intimately, but once they spend time with me they really love me and want to be with me. I carried the decision that I was a disappointment as a woman for thirty-six years. My parents were disappointed momentarily, and I was vulnerable and accepted that as my Personal Lie. By the time I met Jeff, I had been involved with the Loving Relationships Training for five years, and most of me knew I was a surprisingly wonderful woman. Then this conception/birth memory I had in New York pushed me into really accepting how wanted and loved I was.

You are probably wondering what the conception of our relationship was like. It was really no big deal. That's probably the way both our own conceptions were. (My parents were planning for a boy, and Jeff's parents wanted a child to keep Jeff's dad out of the war.) The first time Jeff and I saw each other was in April of 1985. Sondra Ray and I were leading a reunion completion evening for the Loving Relationships Training in Los Angeles. Jeff came that night with his girlfriend to learn about the LRT. Sondra and I immediately noticed Jeff and commented "Who is that—he is really great looking!"

He confessed later that his thoughts about me were, "What great legs she has," and, "I bet she never does any house work." By the way, I do housework sometimes, and I hate it.

Jeff did his first LRT in June with his girlfriend, after which they broke up. Nine months to the day after they broke up, we started our intimate relationship, on March 13, 1986. For six months before that we were becoming very close friends.

Jeff took a wet rebirthing training I led, and I chose him to be my rebirther. I saw him as being handsome, sensitive, strong, supportive, loving, extremely funny, and somewhat macho but sweet. These were all the qualities I wanted in a man for an intimate relationship. I figured that if he rebirthed me, I might get closer to attracting that kind of man. I never expected that Jeff would be the one. We both thought the other one was safe. Jeff was recovering from his last relationship, and I had a two-month relationship going on which had been interrupted by the guy going to Africa for two months. We were both quite surprised at how close we had become. There was no thought of having sex with each other.

We rebirthed each other weekly, and started talking on the phone regularly. We went to parties together around Christmas and New Year's. We found ourselves sharing everything with each other. He would drive me to LRT

Previews in San Diego, Orange County and Santa Barbara. We were always going on long drives and pouring our hearts out to each other.

The beauty of our relationship was how unexpected it was; neither of us had planned to fall in love with the other. Love came very gradually. Each of us was conceived for reasons that were at odds with what we were. We each had to gradually create our parents adoring us. That was what our relationship was like.

One day Jeff was rebirthing me and I was confessing to him how many men I had slept with. I said I was trying to prove I was wanted as a woman and not a disappointment. I was trying to prove on the outside something I didn't know inside myself. At that point Jeff said he could never be with a woman like that. It certainly was a surprise when we did surrender to each other intimately.

New Year's Eve, 1986, Jeff and I went to a party. At midnight we kissed after having had a few drinks. That was the first time I had the thought that maybe this relationship was more than just a friendship. People were commenting everywhere we went what a great couple we were. We always laughed and said we were just friends. Everyone else knew the perfection of our relationship before we recognized it.

On January 12, 1986 the man I thought I had a relationship with returned from Africa. We had a difficult time reconnecting and ended our intimate relationship on January 16th. January 16th was Jeff's birthday, and I was supposed to rebirth him for his birthday. I was very upset about breaking up the other relationship that I had thought was right for me. Jeff consented to rebirth me on his birthday. He wet rebirthed me and I started to cry under the water. I came up and said, "I wonder if I will ever find a man who can handle all my love. . ." Jeff was very touched by this and later shared with me that he had felt he could handle all my love. He had always felt that women didn't appreciate or love him enough after a certain period of time. He knew he wanted a lot of love, affection, and attention, since as an only child he was used to a lot of love. He was really the perfect man for me.

At one point I sat down and talked to myself about why I wasn't attracting men who wanted to be as intimate as I thought I wanted to be. I admitted to myself my own fear of intimacy. I had always attracted men who had a lot of fear of intimacy. I thought this was their case. However, when I admitted my 100% responsibility for choosing relationships that only got so close, I recognized my own fear. Then I was able to attract what I had thought I always wanted—someone who really loved me deep to the core. Someone who loved everything about me, totally appreciated me, and completely recognized that I was a "surprisingly wonderful woman".

At first when Jeff wanted to be intimate with me I didn't think he was the right one for me. Actually he wanted to be with me sexually because he had been celibate for nine months, and he wanted to be sexual with a woman he felt safe with. He felt safe with me, but didn't think at that time he wanted a relationship with me.

I knew if I was with him sexually we would probably end up in a relationship. I had the pattern of attracting men who thought they just wanted sex with me, then fell in love with me. This relates to my conception and birth decisions. I wanted to make sure that if I was intimate with Jeff, it was for the right reasons, and not because of my usual patterns or being horny. We were very close, and I didn't want to lose the friendship for a couple of nights of sex. I also wanted to come from choice; knowing I wanted to be with him.

I started thinking about all the things I loved about Jeff. The list was very, very long. He supported me 100% in everything I did. He really listened to me. He was easy to talk to. He knew a lot about things I was interested in. He was a lot of fun and really funny. He was very handsome. I love tall men, and he is 6′3″. He was sweet to my children. He loved animals. He had three dogs and I had two dogs and three cats. I liked doing the same things he did. He loved to eat and so did I. He was a great cook. He loved to drive me wherever I wanted to go. He always made me feel good. He was a total gentleman. He opened doors for me and walked on the street side of the sidewalk just like my dad. He liked sports and he cussed. The list went on and on—actually I had written a description of my ideal relationship with a man. On January 3, 1985, Jeff had 98% of everything on the list.

Why didn't I want to be with this man? I could only think of a few things. He was having more financial problems then I was, and at that time I was in debt. He seemed to have a very heavy death urge. Everyone in his family had died. His step-father died fifteen years ago. His mom, dad and favorite dog had all died three years before, within six months of each other. He seemed to really be sinking into that. We actually got closer when my dog, Midnight, was dying of cancer.

Twice Jeff had spent the night and we had cuddled; he was very warm and I really liked that. I am wide awake in the mornings—I jump right out of my bed. He was unconscious—I couldn't talk or relate to him. He was incoherent till he had three or four cups of coffee. This bothered me a lot. Also, he smoked, which should have bothered me but didn't. I saw that there were a lot more reasons to be with Jeff than not. By making excuses I saw I could be avoiding a wonderful relationship.

Jeff always asked me what I wanted. He really was interested in giving me what I wanted. It scared me that I had finally found someone who wanted to give me what I wanted sexually. Before we were intimate, he would ask me what I liked and wanted. I wouldn't tell him because I didn't want him to get that close to me. Complaining that men never gave me what I wanted was what I was used to. Here was a man who wanted to give me exactly what I wanted, and I was pushing him away.

Everyone who has made decisions like mine does the same things. If we feel unwanted we are addicted to proving that we are unwanted by choosing men who don't want us. We will push away the ones who want us. If they want us, there must be something wrong with them. Well, I saw Jeff had a lot more right with him than what I judged as wrong. My judgments were merely my justification for pushing him away.

I discussed with him the things that bothered me. I knew the money issue was ridiculous, because when you are loved and you have great sex, you always make more money. I knew that both our money cases would be healed by our love and sexual energy. Sex is creative energy. So the more sexy you are, the more money you create. I knew this from the past. When I had good sex, I made more money.

We discussed the unconscious death urge issue. I suggested that maybe cold water rebirthing would help. Cold water rebirthing helps to release the death urge by releasing fear. Also you breathe very fast, so you can warm up your body. This helps to get rid of anesthesia stored in the body. Jeff's mom was heavily anesthetized at his birth, so that created some of his unconsciousness in the morning. I am a real advocate of cold water rebirthing after people have done at least eight or nine private rebirthing sessions with the same rebirther. My experience is that it helps people to fear forward.

Fear is just the anticipation of something bad happening. We all have some fear of getting into cold water and having it be uncomfortable. The first time I did a cold water rebirth, as I put my head in the water my immediate thought was, "If I do this I will die." I came up, shared it, and then moved through it. I never consciously thought I had a death urge. However, I dated a mortician for eighteen months. So of course, I was dealing with my unconscious death urge like anyone else. I dated the mortician right after I left my eight-year marriage. My marriage was so dead, the mortician really seemed alive to me by comparison. I was taking the LRT and getting rebirthed at the time I was dealing with him. He became my response column to my aliveness. When I chose life 100%, I left the mortician behind.

Cold water rebirthing is very exhilarating and really makes you feel alive and conscious in your body. Jeff did a cold/hot water rebirthing weekend I led. He decided to do cold water rebirthing everyday for awhile. He did it almost every day for about six months. He had immediate results. He now wakes up really clear and conscious, even at 6 or 7 a.m. He usually gets out of bed before me.

He also stopped smoking. I actually used to enjoy his smoking because his favorite time to smoke was after making love. He looked very sexy. And when he lit up at other times, I found myself getting turned on.

After two months of saying "no" to sex, it seemed right and I surrendered to Jeff's love. He made such great shifts in the things I was concerned about that I decided to let him want me. I stopped resisting him. I can't tell you how glad I am that I gave into my divine self instead of my response column.

Sex just gets better and better because we trust each other. We communicate and clear daily. We ask for what we want. We started the relationship very consciously. We saw the things that could be potential problems, and we cleared them first. In the past I rushed into sex and it didn't work. I am grateful for our patience, and for the fact that we pushed through to have what we both really wanted.

In the couple's intensive, couples acknowledged us for the joy we had around each other all the time. The joy we have in taking drives together, walking on the beach, eating a great meal, collecting rocks or just holding hands, is the same joy we always have when we make love.

Conception Case Histories

This section shows how specific conception situations affect adult sexuality. The conception situations discussed are:

1. The conception was a mistake, illegitimate or an accident.
2. The conception was unplanned or unwanted by one or both parents.
3. At conception, one or both parents wanted a baby of the opposite sex.
4. At conception, the new being felt guilty of intruding on his or her parents' life.
5. At conception, the father was drunk and having affairs.
6. At conception, the baby was wanted for the wrong reasons.
7. At conception, sex was a duty for the mother.
8. At conception, the father was angry in general, and angry about the conception.

The Conception Was a Mistake, Illegitimate or an Accident

LISA

Conception description .... My conception was a mistake, but very exciting. Also, my mother was raped when I was in the womb.

How my conception affects my sexuality .... I feel I have to be alone. I am always having sex with the wrong man. It is always a mistake. I feel men destroy my life. I have been a prostitute, which makes me really feel that sex is always wrong and a mistake. I feel guilty about this.

EVA

Conception description .... My conception was both exciting and forbidden. I feel guilty about my conception.

How my conception affects my sexuality .... I feel guilty about sex. I don't give myself as much pleasure as I would like to. I am afraid to let go and relax.

ANNETTE

Conception description .... I was unplanned, unwanted and an accident.

How my conception affects my sexuality .... I like brief and spontaneous affairs. I like seduction and leisurely love-making. I am uncomfortable with commitment. I like illegitimate affairs. I have always had a fascination with prostitution. I once was a call girl in Germany for two months.

MARILYN

Conception description .... My mother was sixteen when I was conceived. I was unplanned and an accident. My father was older. They got married after they discovered she was pregnant. My mother felt like a prostitute.

How my conception affects my sexuality .... If I really go for it in sex I'll be a prostitute. Getting married makes sex legitimate. You get what you want with sex if you get married.

PETER

Conception description . . . . My parents were at a party and my mom was flirting with other men. My father wanted to marry my mom but she didn't want to get married. Mom got pregnant after the party. She wanted to abort me but my father talked her into getting married instead.

How my conception affects my sexuality . . . . I choose women who are withholding sexually and not readily available to me. If a woman wants me, I get scared and want to run away.

The Conception Was Unplanned or Unwanted by One or Both Parents

ALLISON

Conception description . . . . My father was sure he wanted to conceive me, but my mother wasn't. She wasn't because when I was born, she gave up her career.

How my conception affects my sexuality . . . . I have most of my life known a terror of getting pregnant, and felt somehow that sex is dangerous, and leads to a kind of death. I totally suppressed these thoughts by being on the pill, but now, in trying to conceive a child myself, they are surfacing. Since I stopped taking the pill, I have been pregnant 3 times. So the thought that pregnancy leads to death has been acted out so far with the fetuses. I guess I'm still afraid that if the child survives, I'll die.

JEANIE

Conception description . . . . My mom had two other children. I was number three, and I felt I was the straw that broke the camel's back. I was not wanted. I felt tremendous anger and hurt from my mother. I perceived and manifested this in the womb, and in the outside world after I was born.

How my conception affects my sexuality . . . . I had a hook-up between sex and anger, and love and anger. I felt that I was not wanted, for me, sexually by a partner.

My partners had to be very angry in order to love sex with me. I also perceived that I was too much for my partners, and wanted sex too much, but never got it. I perceived men, and life in general, as being too much, and that I hurt people. I felt guilty at just being anywhere.

BETSY

Conception description . . . . I've never really thought about this before, but I find it does fit in with my feeling that sex is dirty. My mother was an art student. My father was working on his Masters in voice. The two families knew each other, and were apparently both unusual in that all my grandparents were college graduates. Education has always been important to my adopted parents too. My father didn't know of my existence, so I gather this was not a long-standing relationship. It may even have been a one-night fling.

How my conception affects my sexuality . . . . I have always felt that sex was a duty I performed so that I might get attention and love. The sooner the actual penetration was over, the better. Being illegitimate makes me feel like I was the unwanted product of something dirty and ugly. I have often had sex in secretive, out-of-the-way places. When I had sex where I lived, I felt intruded upon.

I feel out of touch with my birth. I know nothing of the actual birth except that my adopted parents were told that it was "natural." I'm not sure what that means. This was in 1948, so I assume it was whatever was routine then.

When I have sex, I separate my head from my body and go through the motions. Since my marriage this has happened less and less, but I used to re-decorate rooms or make shopping lists in my head during sex. I was simply on automatic from the neck down. The more used I felt, the deader I would become. Since my mother stayed with me for a few weeks after my birth, I probably had time to bond with her. Then she left. Men always left me, or sometimes, I left them.

JOHN

Conception description . . . . My folks conceived me two months before they got married. Mom says she would not have married Dad if she hadn't gotten pregnant. Or rather, to be exact, she says she was testing whether she could have kids with Dad before they got married.

How my conception affects my sexuality . . . . This really brings up survival issues for me. I have to have women, or rather sex, in order to "get married" to life so to speak. In order for me to live fully, happily and be complete, I need to either talk about sex, come on strong, or something. That is my negative thought based on the issue my mom had: "Can I have kids with Yuchi [my dad] or not. If not, should I even marry him?!?!"

When I do have sex, which is not real often, it's great. I'm confused, which comes up in how women perceive me. On the one hand, Mom says I'm a child of true love, but on the other hand, she might not have married Dad if they could not have had babies. Why put this burden on me even before I was born?

MICHAEL

Conception description . . . . Mother wanted a girl. Not wanted by father.

How my conception affects my sexuality . . . . Suppressed male energy. As a child I was a loner.

During high school I had girl friends—usually long term and serious relationships. I got very depressed when they left—felt totally rejected. They represented my father. I would see girls who wanted me—they represented my mother, whom I was angry at. I blamed her for my father leaving—incest pattern—I suppose.

I've always had the thought that I don't completely know how to be a man because my father wasn't there for me. The thought implies I still need him.

KATHIE

Conception description . . . . Coming into the world unwanted and an embarrassment to my mother did not create a very secure feeling in me. When their first reaction to me was "Yuk, what an ugly baby", that dipped the bottom out of the security.

How my conception affects my sexuality . . . . I never was sure how I looked, and spent a great deal of time and energy making sure no one would find out how yucky and ugly I was.

JANIS

Conception description .... I was unplanned. My mother had had her tubes tied prior to my conception.

How my conception affects my sexuality .... "I don't know if I've done the right thing being here". This thought is very strong when I commence having sex. I feel like an intruder—like I shouldn't be there, that my partners would rather be with someone else. I hate planning to have sex—I like it to be spontaneous.

KATHLEEN

Conception description .... I had the thought at the moment of conception, "I don't belong here, something is terribly wrong because this is a loveless, unconscious consummation. They don't love each other, therefore they must not love me."My father actually told my mother that if I had been a boy, he would have taken me to raise.

How my conception affects my sexuality .... I concluded that I was unlovable, unwanted and unconscious. That is how I have perceived my relationships to be. Hot sex, but no intimate love.

I made the decision that I was not good enough as a woman because my parents did not want me. So I attract men who are incapable of intimacy, emotionally aloof, and who can only relate to me on a sexual level. I overcompensate for my feeling of inadequacy by trying to be as sexually pleasing as possible. So I end up in a fucking relationship rather than a loving relationship. I can only reach orgasm by sexual fantasy, when I'm high from smoking pot, in "kinky" sex, or with "wild" men.

At Conception, One or Both Parents Wanted a Baby of the Opposite Sex

HARRIET

Conception description .... My father wanted a boy.

How my conception affects my sexuality .... I don't feel safe in an intimate relationship with a man, because they really don't want me as a woman.

I have the thought that I am nothing special. I often try to overcompensate for this thought by overachieving sexually.

JEFF

Conception description .... My parents wanted a girl. My mom hated sex. Sex hurt my mom.

How my conception affects my sexuality .... I was often teased for being too cute for a boy. I should have been a girl. I am gay. My mother was hurt when she found out I was gay. I have been hurt and abused sexually in past relationships. I fear that I am not wanted as a man, but wanted as a sex object.

LINDA

Conception description .... I was conceived to carry on the family name—they wanted a boy. There was also a fear that I would be retarded, like my mother's sister.

How my conception affects my sexuality .... I feel retarded in the area of sexuality. I don't feel lovable or wanted as a woman.

DANA

Conception description .... I was not planned or wanted as a girl. I was conceived when my parents didn't have much money.

How my conception affects my sexuality .... I feel that I am too much as a woman sexually. I want to be taken care of by a man in a relationship. I feel wrong and guilty, because what I want sexually and financially is too much for a man to handle.

ELLEN

Conception description .... My parents wanted a boy. At my conception, my father was drunk and my mother denied her sexuality.

How my conception affects my sexuality .... I deny my sexuality. I have pain and suffering hooked up with sex. I have spent my whole life denying that I am a woman.

At Conception, the New Being Felt Guilty of Intruding on His or Her Parents' Life.

PETER

Conception description .... My parents had a really romantic life. I feel I held them back from doing what they really wanted to do.

How my conception affects my sexuality .... I always feel guilty in sex. I don't feel worthy of all the love and attention I am getting from my partner. I push people away because I feel guilty and unworthy of their love.

SHARON

Conception description .... I always felt that my father met my mother's needs sexually but was not there for her emotionally. I'm also getting that there was some confusion about monogamy on my father's part.

My conception was honest and open, and I have always felt that about my sexuality.

What I feel I got from my mother at conception was sexual guilt. Feeling guilty because she knew when they were having sex in order to conceive a child, that she really didn't want children, but gave up her power to my father because he did want a family.

How my conception affects my sexuality .... Up until I moved to Georgia, I created men who met my needs sexually but were unavailable for me emotionally. After I moved, I created men who were not available or satisfying sexually either.

Like my father, I'm feeling confusion about monogamy.

I have always been open and honest about my preferences in sex, and my pure enjoyment of sex. But, like my mother, there is a part of me that gives up my power in order to please men.

I have created for myself either extremely pleasurable sex, a little on the wild side, or experiences that were very bad, that made me feel powerless, guilt-ridden, or with a large dose of disapproval. From my guilt I have created sexual health problems such as VD, cystitis, vaginal infections, and pelvic inflammatory disease. Also, the guilt created a case of rape.

The rape occurred within earshot of my mother, and I had so much fear of her disapproval that I didn't cry out, but did as she had done at my conception—gave in. (The rape was by someone I knew, so I knew I wouldn't be hurt physically.) So, on moving to Georgia, I tried to find a person to stay with who would not satisfy me sexually. I covered myself with fat so as to be unattractive so I could be monogamous and safe.

But that didn't work because I created a relationship with someone who was married. He was very attracted to me sexually and as a person. So the choice was living with an available but unsatisfying sexual partner, or having a sexual partner who was satisfying but already was in a different primary relationship.

At Conception, the Father Was Drunk and Having Affairs With Other Women

MICHAEL

Conception description .... My father drank a lot, and he was having affairs with other women at the time I was conceived. My mother thought that my father really wanted someone other than her.

How my conception affects my sexuality .... I often feel that my partner really wants someone else sexually.

At Conception, the Baby Was Wanted for the Wrong Reasons

KAREN

Conception description .... I was wanted and planned by my mother to keep my father in the relationship. He left anyway.

How my conception affects my sexuality .... I have a fear of a pregnancy I don't want, which prevents me from enjoying sex. I am not there and available for sex in the same way my father was not there and available to me.

SCOTT

Conception description .... I was very wanted and planned. There had been several miscarriages before me. My grandmother died when my mother was pregnant with me. I was named for my grandmother. I feel I wanted to get rid of my grandmother so I would have my mother's full attention.

How my conception affects my sexuality . . . . I always feel responsible for fulfilling other people's expectations. In sex, I feel that I am not fully there. I feel I will either hurt or kill my partner. I pull in women sexually and then I push them away. I think that if I deaden myself sexually, then my partner can live.

At Conception, Sex Was a Duty for the Mother

MARGORETTE

Conception description . . . . I feel that my mother felt sex was a duty. You had to do it if you were a woman. She also felt it was sinful.

How my conception affects my sexuality . . . . I feel I can't get what I want sexually, I can't get pleasure.

VIVIENNE

Conception description . . . . My mother had sex as her duty to my father and she was scared. She had resistance to sex—she felt that it was disgusting and dirty. My parents wanted a boy.

How my conception affects my sexuality . . . . I have resistance to men and their bodies. I don't feel wanted as a woman by men. I can't let go in sex. I think my boyfriend would be better off with another woman. I am not a pleasure to men or myself sexually.

JULIE

Conception description . . . . My mother's thought at my conception was that it is only OK for men to have pleasure.

How my conception affects my sexuality . . . . In sex, I have to get it over with fast, so the man has pleasure but I don't. I don't feel safe getting the pleasure I want.

At Conception, Father Angry in General, and Angry about the Conception

LOUISE

Conception description . . . . My father was angry when I was conceived.

How my conception affects my sexuality . . . . I have a lot of anger at men, and I attract angry men in sexual relationships. I have gained a lot of weight, which I know has to do with my anger at men.

NIEJA

Conception description . . . . There was a lot of anger and frustration.

How my conception affects my sexuality . . . . I am either angry at my partner and suppress it, and then I cannot feel anything at all, or I am angry and express it, and then I can really feel excited when making love.

CHAPTER 2

Womb

Nine-Month Honeymoon Period

I AM SITTING writing this chapter at Zaca Lake at a spiritual retreat with Sondra Ray, Fredric Lehrman, and thirty-three other people. The setting of the lake has brought up for many of us the experience of being in the womb. It is a beautiful, peaceful, green, natural lake surrounded on all sides by mountains and pine trees. The road into the lake is a very narrow dirt road, very much like a birth canal. It is seven miles long. Being here for me brings up the peace and tranquility I must have felt in the womb. All the chanting, meditating, and studying of *A Course In Miracles* that we have done all week, plus the peace, harmony and serenity of the physical environment has inspired me to write this chapter.

The amazing thing about all of this is that Jeffrey Baker and I had our nine month anniversary of our intimate relationship on the day we drove up the seven mile road to Zaca Lake. As rebirthers, we laughed and joked about the significance of our nine months together and how the seven mile road reminded us of a birth canal. We also knew that our relationship was going to change, but at that time we had no idea how. Nine months always signifies rebirth, birth, and change.

Jeff had only driven me up to the lake and was leaving two days later. He had not planned to participate in the week-long spiritual retreat. The day that Jeff left I went through my whole birth in a rebirth which I will describe in another chapter.

For now I want to get into the feelings of what the first nine months of a relationship represents and how it is like being in the womb.

The womb is warm, safe, nurturing, and all encompassing. There is nothing else out there for the baby—just the womb, the connection to the mother through the umbilical cord, the walls of the womb and the warm gentle motion of the water.

I'm sitting on a balcony overlooking the lake—the sun is coming up to warm the water. There is a cloud of smoke over the water—floating very lightly above the water. It is quite still and everything is moving very slowly. There is classical music in the background. Even the ducks on the lake are floating at peace and at one with the motion of the lake. The feeling is that everything is handled and it is so easy and pleasurable to just be here and exist. Everything is in sync with everything else around it. All the ducks are swimming in the same rhythm toward the center of the lake to the music. Fredric is playing Impromptu in D-Flat by Schubert. Impromptu is perfect for the spontaneous, carefree movements of the womb.

As I experience this, I now know what it felt like in the womb. I can see myself being one of the small little ducks on the huge lake, having not a care in the world, just floating around experiencing the warmth, space and motion of the lake. In the beginning that is what we felt like: at-one-with and not in opposition to anything, just floating and being in every breath.

In the beginning of a relationship we are like that. We are in bliss with each other; there is no one else out there. All we are interested in is knowing and exploring each part of each other slowly and lovingly, just as the baby lovingly explores its environment. Sometimes you never want to get out of bed. You want to explore—to explore every part of each other's body and to get to feel that harmony and at-one feeling with your partner, the same way you lovingly explored each part of the womb.

In the first nine months of our relationship we re-experienced the bliss of our womb memories, the peace, joy and love.

Intimacy, sex and love bring up all the memories of this peaceful womb. We all start out like this, after two or three months, things might change in our intimate experience. Whatever happened when we were in the womb will be re-experienced in the relationship. The baby feels everything that is happening outside of the womb. After the initial blissful exploring stage, our relationship might change according to what was happening outside of the womb and what decisions the baby was making about what was happening with his or her parents. Often relationships change or end after nine months because there were dramatic changes and decisions made at this time that still effect us now in our relationships.

Some of us might have felt wonderful for the first six months, but then things seemed to change. This might be the time that the intimate relationship changes. It is important to look back on your intimate relationships: is there a pattern of time when the relationship ends or dramatically changes from peace and harmony to more struggle. Was it three months, six months or nine months?

I know with my relationship with Jeff the first nine months represented that idea of exploration, of getting to know and feel each other. Especially in the beginning it felt like nothing else mattered but being with him. We both were the center of each other's universe. We spent as much time together as possible and when we were not together physically, we shared on the phone everything that was happening to us throughout the day. We were blending, learning how to be totally at one with each other. We were merging ourselves into each other as we merged with the womb. There was no struggle or desire to rock the boat.

As the nine months womb experience comes to an end, the womb becomes more constricted, the baby gets bigger, and there is a decision made—it is time to change, it is time to leave here and come out. This has been wonderful, but something must be even better out there, because it is getting harder to move, and feel free. It is time to share myself with the world.

How this could look sexually is that in the beginning sex could be totally uninhibited, blissful, exploring every crevice, and part of each other. There's lots of energy and movement. Then sex might become more boring. After the initial exploring stage, maybe sex even becomes restrictive. Often thoughts come up of No Exit Terror, a feeling of having to get out of here, and severe claustrophobia.

I have had lovers who have jumped up right after sex and opened the windows. I had one relationship where after about eight months he could not even lie close to me. He would go to sleep at the opposite end of the bed. His feet would be up at my face. He was a transverse lie, which means that he was lying across his mother's stomach when he was in the womb. He could not get out, he was lying in the wrong direction to get out of the birth canal. Toward the ninth month of our relationship he became claustrophobic and usually got up at four or five in the morning and went home. He was experiencing NO EXIT TERROR. He couldn't get out of the womb and he felt suffocated and trapped. A caesarean was necessary to rescue him. So in the intimate relationship with me he was re-experiencing the same feelings of suffocation and feeling trapped. The only way he could feel better was to leave.

What we all do in the beginning of our relationships is experience bliss, harmony, and at-one feelings. Our mind then strives for familiarity, so we recreate exactly what happened to us in the womb. If we got claustrophobic we might have to leave or we might create lots of struggle in our relationships so we will get kicked out of the relationship.

The way to change this would be to become aware of what your womb experience was like. Often in rebirthing people re-experience being in the womb in order to understand it better. You could also do the same thing that I just did. Go to a lake or peaceful place and meditate on what the womb felt like for you.

Look back on your relationships and try to remember what happened during the first nine months. If you have created something you don't like over and over again you can change it. The first step in changing a pattern you don't want is to recognize or gain an awareness of what you are continually recreating.

The next step is to recognize your addiction to this pattern. This addiction can be like any other addiction to alcohol, drugs, food, or overeating. Once you admit the addiction and recognize the payoffs you are receiving for keeping the addiction you can choose out by saying "no" to the pattern. Usually people indulge in the pattern one last time so they are really sick of it, so that saying "no" becomes easier and easier and eventually you will say goodbye to the pattern forever. It's important to understand that change is safe so that you will choose out of the patterns that no longer work for you. Just as we chose out of the womb because it doesn't serve us any longer, we can choose out of our negative patterns that no longer give us what we want.

Affirmations for the Womb Period

1. Change is safe.
2. Intimacy and sex are safe.
3. I can move and breathe when I am intimate.
4. Pleasure follows bliss.
6. There is always something new to explore.
7. Sex is always a new, never-ending, exciting adventure.
8. Being close is safe.
9. The next step is even better and more exciting.
10. Decisions are safe and easy.
11. Change is always very exciting.
12. The sexual honeymoon is never over.

CHAPTER 3

Birth

How Birth Affects Us Sexually

OUR BIRTH SCRIPT contains all the decisions that we made about life at our birth. This script runs us in life, especially whenever we are going through change. We have this automatic pilot that we switch on whenever change comes up that makes us recreate our Birth Script. No matter how terrible it was, we survived our Birth Script. We made the decision that in order to survive we have to recreate our birth scenario. If the birth script has pain, struggle, guilt, hurting your mother or being hurt, drugs, forceps, or separation, we relive this sequence of events over and over again in our intimate relationships.

In the earlier chapter on the womb or honeymoon sexual period we talked about how great sex is in the beginning. For the first six to nine months usually people in an intimate relationship are totally consumed with each other. There is nothing else out there except their partner. Then around nine months it gets claustrophobic and the "let me out of here" or "no exit terror syndrome" is relived. The partner who once created total bliss and love by wanting to be with you every minute now all of a sudden is suffocating you with all their love. Time patterns really play a part in when relationships end. The nine month time period always creates a dramatic change in the relationship.

As I mentioned earlier Jeff and I were separated for a week exactly at our nine month anniversary. It was time to come out and experience ourselves as separate and unique individuals. Just as at nine months I left my mother, I was compelled to leave Jeff and assert my individuality and independence.

As I go around the world and interview people on how their births effect their sexuality, it's universal no matter what the country, the U.S.A., England,

Sweden, New Zealand, Australia, etc . . . people play out their Birth Scripts sexually with their intimate partners. The interviews I did with people on how their birth effects their sexuality are in subsequent chapters.

I remember one of the first times I made love with Jeff how it re-enacted his whole birth. Jeff was held back at his birth to wait for the doctor who was delivering someone else. When the doctor was ready to deliver him he didn't want to come out. They gave his mother anesthesia and pulled him out with forceps. On this particular night I was cooking dinner and Jeff got turned on and wanted to make love. I made him wait till after we had dinner. This is how I held him back. When I was ready he didn't want to make love. I gave him a drink and a foot rub and this induced him into making love with me. I often feel like I have to induce him into having sex. A drink relaxes him and helps to get him started with sex. I didn't have any drugs at my birth so I always seem more ready to make love.

If you had drugs at your birth you might feel like you need alcohol or drugs to feel comfortable and relaxed enough to have sex.

Since birth is so closely related to sex, sex often triggers all the birth memories. Some women even have orgasms when giving birth if they are relaxed enough. Babies often take on the fear, pleasure, or whatever their mother was feeling at their birth. Often at birth babies feel that they are responsible for the hurt or pain their mother is experiencing. With sex this memory of causing pain to their mother surfaces when people are intimate and having sex with their partners. Often people hold back their sexual aliveness for fear of being hurt or hurting their partner.

If a mother or baby die or come close to death during birth, then sex and death can be hooked up together. Babies who have the cord around their necks at birth may make the decision that the source of their life, the umbilical cord, almost killed them. When they have sex as adults, this memory is triggered. Sex and death can then become associated.

Often people have pain hooked up with sex. There is the birth thought that pain follows pleasure because the womb was pleasurable, then they had pain at birth. Often people will hold back their sexual aliveness and the experience of having pleasure because they expect unconsciously for pain to follow the pleasure.

Many people experience creating an intimate sexual relationship as a struggle. These thoughts usually begin at birth when we felt that we had to struggle to get out of the birth canal. If someone is used to this, they will struggle to create the relationship, but if not struggling there, they will struggle to have sex be the way they want it in their relationship.

If your birth script included a lot of manipulation and intervention from the obstetrician, you will expect your partner to manipulate and control you.

Babies often felt helpless at their birth and that they "can't make it". This is why they needed the obstetrician to help and support them. If this support hurt or was manipulating and controlling, a person will expect to be manipulated and controlled by their intimate partners, but will be angry if they are and even angrier if they aren't. Someone who is forceps or induced will need a partner to gently persuade them to have fun sexually until they change this pattern.

Since I had an issue about being a disappointment as a woman, my first sexual experience was a disappointment. I waited until I was twenty years old. I had been dating my boyfriend for four years, two years of high school and two years of college. We did a lot of passionate making out and doing everything but sexual intercourse. I was really holding out and then when I finally decided to come out sexually I was disappointed. It was the opposite of what I expected. It was terrible. My partner was also disappointed because we had waited so long. My thought was, "This is what everyone makes such a big deal about? What a disappointment!"

My father was disappointed at my birth for seven seconds that I was a girl, then he was happy. I was disappointed that he was disappointed and I held onto the decision that I was a disappointment as a woman. Sex was always disappointing to me because I never had an orgasm until I realized I was a surprisingly wonderful woman. When I integrated that new thought in my body I was then able to have multiple orgasms. Usually when we come out the first thing that is noticed is whether we are a boy or girl. If the reaction we receive is less than excited we become confused about our sexuality. Being confused about our sexuality, or about being a woman or man and not being wanted for the sex that we are, does not lead to a blissful, easy, fun, exciting, pleasurable sex life.

Sexual guilt is another inhibiting factor in having great sex. Sexual guilt often comes from what we call the Infant Guilt Syndrome. As infants we are totally innocent and alive. If our mothers had pain at our births, were drugged, cut for an episiotomy, hemorrhaged or died, we as infants were totally sensitive and took on the guilt of having created that pain for them. It's very logical to think that if we had not been conceived when they had sex then they would not have had pain. We associate our aliveness with their pain.

As grown-ups, we hold back our sexual aliveness for fear of hurting our partner. Or if we are really guilty we could have affairs or leave our sexual partners to hurt them. Since we are addicted to our guilt we find ways to feel our guilt by hurting the ones we love. Guilt demands punishment: when we feel guilty we create punishment. For example, our pain over losing or hurting our partner is a kind of punishment.

Another dimension of guilt can be the case of twins. The one who leaves the womb first may feel guilty for leaving the other behind. In relationships, first twins may re-experience this guilt by leaving their intimate partners. Second twins may find that they are often left by their partners, just as they were left behind at birth.

Over the past two years I have been interviewing people on how their birth effects their sexuality. The next sections are the result of this research.

Birth Case Histories—Birth Types

The following chapter shows how specific birth types and birth situations affect our sexuality.

Birth Types

1. Premature/Incubator
2. Forceps
3. Drugged Birth
4. Cord Around Neck
5. RH Factor Baby
6. Twin
7. Breech Birth
8. Face Presentation
9. Fast Birth
10. Held Back
11. Dry Birth
12. Induced
13. Late Birth
14. Caesarean

Birth Situations

1. The baby was hurt at birth or there was something wrong with the baby.
2. The baby was the wrong sex.
3. The mother was hurt at the birth.
4. The father was not present at the birth.
5. The baby had a long separation from its mother.
6. The baby was stuck.

7. The baby was adopted at birth.
8. There was almost a miscarriage.
9. The mother tried to abort the baby.
10. The baby was circumcised right after birth.
11. Struggle at birth.

Premature/Incubator

SUSAN

Birth description . . . . My birth was two months premature, drugs and forceps. I was also in an incubator.

How my birth affects my sexuality . . . . I feel I have a wall around me in sex, like I am in the incubator and separate from the experience. I feel that if I let people see me, that I will be too much to handle. My partner will not be able to handle my aliveness and energy: he won't want me if he really sees me.

Another decision I made, because I was an accident and was conceived at a party, was that if you are sexual, you will suffer the consequences of having a baby which is a burden.

NEIL

Birth description . . . . I was five weeks premature. There were lots of babies in the incubator when I was born. Some of the incubator babies had to be put in the hall because it was too crowded. I did not see my mother for three days.

How my birth affects my sexuality . . . . Sex doesn't mean anything to me—it is nonexistent. I feel that I am alone and separate, especially in the area of sexuality.

GENTRY

Birth description . . . . My birth was premature and incubator.

How my birth affects my sexuality . . . . When I was married, I got what I wanted sexually, but I felt I had to get out of there. I jump into relationships quickly and then I regret that I did. I feel that it is dangerous outside, and I have to protect myself from sex.

MIYA

Birth description .... I was one month early. There was an explosion in my house, and I was afraid and wanted to come out. I tried to come out and they stopped me. They finally let me out.

How my birth affects my sexuality .... I always create push-and-pull situations in relationships. Men want me and yet they are afraid of me.

GISELLA

Birth description .... I was two weeks early. My sister and I were very close: we were born the same year. I have had some memories that my sister was supposed to be my twin. When my sister was born, she had a growth that was supposed to be the twin that died. I feel that I am that twin, and that is why I was born so close to my sister.

How my birth affects my sexuality .... I am afraid to be too close, because I have that hooked up with death from when I died as my sister's twin. My dad wanted a boy, so I feel I have to have sex to prove that I am a woman, and wanted as a woman.

BOB

Birth Description .... I was six weeks premature. I was in an incubator for six weeks.

How my birth affects my sexuality .... I feel separate and emotionally self-contained. I feel I can't be vulnerable and open up. I can't depend on anyone to take care of my emotional needs or sexual desires other than myself.

BECKY

Birth description .... My mother was drugged against her will. She had to struggle to live. I was in an incubator for a long time. I was kept separate and quarantined because I had red spots, and they thought I had some disease. I was allergic to breast milk. They took a long time before they found I could drink soy milk without a reaction.

How my birth affects my sexuality . . . . I have a hard time being nourished and receiving affection from my partner. I fear intimacy because I am used to being alone. Being alone seems easier.

Forceps

ANN

Birth description . . . . I was forceps and face presentation. There was a lot of pain for my mother.

How my birth affects my sexuality . . . . In sex, I feel stifled in asking for what I want. I think if I really ask for what I want, I will hurt my partner like I hurt my mother.

CHRISTINA

Birth description . . . . My birth was going fine but they used forceps, and this made me angry.

How my birth affects my sexuality . . . . I feel that men are always trying to get me to have sex their way. Men hurt me and manipulate me in sex.

DANIEL

Birth description . . . . My birth was difficult; one or two days of labor. They used forceps, and I did not want to be born. My mother had a fear of death at my birth, and great pain. I was born in the hospital, and I was only given to my mother for nursing. When I was two days old, my mother almost died, and I was given to another person to be nursed for six weeks.

How my birth affects my sexuality . . . . I have sex connected with pain. I get erections when I read about torture. I made the decision that separation equals survival. I feel more comfortable separate than with people. I lived as a religious celibate for four and a half years. I would meditate and sadism would come up. I could not release it through meditation, so five years ago, at the age of thirty-four, I became attracted to men and became homosexual. I got into sadism with these men, using whips and chains while having sex. I had sex and pleasure hooked up with pain. I could not be with women because of my deep subconscious fear of hurting women like I hurt my mother at birth.

JOHN

Birth description .... I was a forceps delivery. I could not do it on my own or my own way.

How my birth affects my sexuality .... I was a virgin until I was twenty-nine. I have a strong thought that "I can't", which gets activated about having sex. I can't have sex.

JOHN PAUL

Birth description .... I had a long labor. I was a forceps baby. I got stuck at my mother's tailbone. I hurt my mother.

How my birth affects my sexuality .... I feel I hurt women and am also manipulated and controlled by women. I felt disappointed by my first sexual experience.

TERRY

Birth description .... At my birth they used forceps.

How my birth affects my sexuality .... I have to be manipulated to have sex. I am afraid to be vulnerable because of the hurt I felt at my birth.

TORBORG

Birth description .... My mother tried to abort me. They used forceps at my birth. My labor was twenty hours long, and there was a lot of struggle.

How my birth affects my sexuality .... I have a lot of separation feelings tied up with sex. I feel mistrust toward women, and anger that they will hurt me or manipulate me. I feel that sex is associated with struggle and hurt. I try to keep myself from feeling anything sexually. Also, I have the thought that something outside of me will hurt me.

NINA

Birth description .... When I was in the womb, my father beat my mother, mentally and physically. My mother divorced my father before I was born. I had a 48-hour labor. My father was not there. There was a lot of pain for my mother as well as a lot of drugs. I was forceps.

How my birth affects my sexuality .... I don't feel supported by men. Life and intimate relationships are a struggle. I hold back my aliveness to protect myself and my partner from pain. My partner does not please me sexually: he only cares about himself. I feel that I am not good enough to be sexually satisfied.

CHRISTI

Birth description .... Forceps delivery.

How my birth affects my sexuality .... I don't like to initiate sex. I have to have other people pull me out in situations including sex. I get angry when people pull me out even though I expect them to. I also get angry if no one pulls me out. I expect help, and at the same time, I resent getting help. I feel not good enough as a woman. I feel men want me for my male attributes.

BRIAN

Birth description .... I was drugged. There was a lot of pain and struggle. I was pulled out with forceps.

How my birth affects my sexuality .... I make my life hard. I feel like I have to perform sexually to be loved. I don't allow myself pleasure. I bend over backwards to please my partner.

LARRY

Birth description .... Long labor, painful, forceps.

How my birth affects my sexuality .... My partners have to be the obstetrician and initiate sex. Sex is sinful. Orgasm is evil. I hurt my partners.

I had problems getting an erection for my first sexual experience when I was twenty-one.

ERNIE

Birth description . . . . I was a big baby of eleven pounds. They used forceps to pull me out. I hurt my mother because I was so big. She tore. I have scars on my cheeks and the back of my head from the forceps.

How my birth affects my sexuality . . . . I prefer to be seduced. It is too much work to initiate sex. I would rather let my partner do it. I hold back my aliveness out of fear of hurting my partner. I used to be ninety pounds heavier in order to protect myself from intimacy. I recently let go of the weight, and am getting more intimate and closer to my wife.

DALYN

Birth description . . . . I was a transverse lie, with a thirty-six hour labor. I should have been a caesarean. They manually turned me and then pulled me out with forceps. I feel I hurt my mother and myself.

How my birth affects my sexuality . . . . I have confusion with sex. I don't know what direction I am going. I feel disconnected in sex. I feel my aliveness is too much. I feel I have to hold back my sexuality. Sex leads to kids and pregnancy, and I fear pregnancy and kids.

Drugs

VALERIE

Birth description . . . . I was willing to be an easy birth with no struggle. I had a short labor, and then they heavily drugged my mother anyway.

How my birth affects my sexuality . . . . I anticipate sex to be great, and then I get bored with it. I feel like I need to be seduced into having sex: I feel as though I am drugged out or numbed out. I like my partner to be the initiator. I am addicted to the orgasm. Like birth, the orgasm is the highlight of sex. I don't like the middle of sex—it feels too controlled. I am waiting for the orgasm to come.

SUSIE

Birth description . . . . My birth was going fine and it was interrupted with anesthesia.

How my birth affects my sexuality . . . . In sex I go unconscious. I always interrupt it with business—thinking about calls, etc.. There is always a struggle to get sex started, but once I get started, when I am not going unconscious, I enjoy it.

NANCY

Birth description . . . . My mother was given drugs which stopped the natural progression of my birth. I was not born until the next day.

How my birth affects my sexuality . . . . In sex, the energy gets stopped somehow and it takes a long time to get it right again.

BEN

Birth description . . . . My mother was not there emotionally or physically at my birth—she was heavily drugged and out to lunch. I felt separate from my mother, like we were not in this thing together. The midwife was rough.

How my birth affects my sexuality . . . . I feel that is better and safer to be alone. Also, I was from an orthodox Jewish family where marriages were arranged, or different from what I wanted. My first date wasn't until I was twenty-four. I feel unwanted as a man by women, as I felt unwanted by my mother.

CAROLINE

Birth description . . . . I had a long labor and I was drugged. I felt out of my body and numbed. My mother wanted a boy, and my father felt threatened by a baby. It hurt when I tried to get out.

How my birth affects my sexuality . . . . I feel my aliveness causes me and other people pain. I feel numb and out of my body when having sex. I am frightened of letting go sexually—I feel that if I really let go in sex like I let go at birth, I will be hurt.

MATTS

Birth description .... At my birth I was drugged.

How my birth affects my sexuality .... I can't give pleasure to women. Other men can pleasure women but I can't. I will hurt women if I try to pleasure them.

PAUL

Birth description .... I was anesthetized for twelve hours.

How my birth affects my sexuality .... I feel anesthetized in my intimate relationships. I feel out of touch with my feelings. I feel not good enough when women criticize me. I feel I can't please women. I feel no matter what I do sexually, it is not enough to please my partner.

Cord Around Neck

RAPHEAL

Birth description .... I was a fast birth—I was delivered in fifteen minutes. I was held back because I was coming too fast, and I had the cord around my neck. I was a blue baby. I wanted to nurse, but didn't get to.

How my birth affects my sexuality .... I always try to make sex fast and easy for my partner. I feel I can't get what I want from women sexually. I hurt women, and women try to kill me. I hold back my sexual energy so I won't hurt women, and women won't kill me.

INNES

Birth description .... My birth was a disappointment because I was a girl. My parents, especially my father, wanted a boy. I had the cord around my neck. There was a struggle for me to live. My father was the obstetrician who delivered me, and he hurt me. My sister was jealous when I was born.

How my birth affects my sexuality . . . . If I really let go in sex, I will die. I have to hold back my energy or aliveness so I won't hurt my partner like I hurt my mother. I create women being jealous, and wanting the man I am sexual with. The men I love hurt me.

LOITA

Birth description . . . . I had a terrible birth. I had the cord around my neck two times. The waters broke twenty-four hours before I was born, so I was a dry birth. I stayed late in the womb, and didn't want to come out: this hurt my mother.

How my birth affects my sexuality . . . . I am always extremely irritated by my boyfriends, and I create lots of conflicts in my sexual relationships. I have the thought that I cause pain to the ones I love, and I had better leave the man I love so I don't cause him pain. Throughout the weekend, I tried to leave my boyfriend.

GINNELLA

Birth description . . . . My mother's first baby was a boy who lived for only eight hours. My mother was scared about sex because that leads to pregnancy, which leads to birth, which could lead to death. My birth was delayed three weeks. My mother was so worried about my birth that I did not want to come out. I had the cord around my neck three times. My mother tried to stop me from coming out because she had so much fear. I hurt my mother because I was so late and I got so big: I was too much.

How my birth affects my sexuality . . . . I do not enjoy sex with my husband. The only time I enjoy sex is if I have drugs, which relaxes me. I don't want to be here, and I feel something is wrong with me, especially in the area of sex. Sometimes I feel that if I really let go sexually, I could die.

RUSSELL

Birth description . . . . I did not want to be born and I tried to avoid birth. They induced me, and I had the cord around my neck, and I was a dry birth.

How my birth affects my sexuality . . . . I am terrified to take the initiative in sex. I wait for someone else to take the initiative, because I think what I am sexually is evil. I suppress my sexuality because it will hurt or kill my partner or myself.

ROSEMARY

Birth description .... I had a normal, very slow birth, and I had the cord around my neck.

How my birth affects my sexuality .... I have death and sex related. I hold back sexuality, and I get very depressed around sexual issues. Sex for me is associated with pain. When I was seventeen, I wanted to get rid of my virginity. The experience was extremely painful.

RH Baby

PAULETTE

Birth description .... I had a drug birth, and I was a RH baby. I needed transfusions at my birth to live. My father wanted a boy.

How my birth affects my sexuality .... I look to men to validate my femininity through sex. Sex with men is like the transfusion: I need it to feel alive. I also have the thought that there is something wrong with me sexually. My ex-husband wanted a buddy, not a woman. Men reject me for being a woman. I also feel rejected by men sexually.

Twin

LOIS

Birth description .... I was a twin and premature. I was the second twin. I feel I don't deserve to live.

How my birth affects my sexuality .... I always feel wrong sexually. I feel I don't deserve to have sex the way I want it.

MAX

Birth description .... I was the first-born of twins. My mother had a lot of fear at our birth, because her mother had died at her birth. I felt like I could hurt or kill someone by being born. My twin was a girl.

How my birth affects my sexuality . . . . Because I have a twin sister, I feel close to the feminine aspect of myself, as well as feeling close to women. I feel close to women, but at the same time they make me feel claustrophobic. I feel that I abandoned my sister and left her behind. I often leave women behind in relationships. I feel evil and naughty. I had incest with my sisters, and I always draw in two women in relationship.

OLAF

Birth description . . . . My parents wanted one baby—I was the second twin. They didn't know I was there until I came out. My mother was drugged at my birth.

How my birth affects my sexuality . . . . I feel invisible and always second in relationships; I put my partner first. I go unconscious if my partner takes the initiative in sex. Then she becomes uninterested and ignores what I want. I feel that I don't get what I want sexually. I don't deserve what I want because I was unwanted and invisible. My needs sexually seem invisible.

Breech Birth

PATRICK

Birth description . . . . I was a breech birth that they manually turned in the womb. I felt intruded on when they turned me. I had drugs before I came out, then I was separated from my mother.

How my birth affects my sexuality . . . . I don't like touch. I developed a "hands-off attitude". I don't like when people touch me. I feel manipulated in sex. I feel like I am having sex for my partner instead of for myself sometimes.

SAM

Birth description . . . . Breech; induced, then held back; long labor; mother lost lots of blood; not breastfed, collicky, threw up all the time; separated from mother for two days; mother depressed.

How my birth affects my sexuality . . . . Since I hurt my mother, I hurt my partner. I pinch her arm or am clumsy. It takes me a long time to get excited.

Someone else has to initiate sex or induce me for sex. Sex is stop and start over. I get excited, then I have to wait for my wife to get excited, and then I'm not excited anymore. I'm excited when my wife isn't, and my wife is excited when I'm not. I feel like I do it wrong because we can't get excited at the same time. My wife was incubator and feels she has to do it alone, so no matter what I do, it doesn't get her excited. We struggle to get started, struggle to get excited, and struggle to be excited at the same time. I'm not spontaneous. I have to be induced or seduced. Then I am angry that I can't do it myself, or be spontaneous.

ROBERT

Birth description .... Breech, anesthesia. Mother was depressed: she wanted a girl.

How my birth affects my sexuality .... I always find something wrong with my partners before they find something wrong with me. I feel guilt about my sexuality. I always feel I will hurt the woman I am with, or she will hurt me. I have anger hooked up with sex. After my first sexual experience at eighteen, I got "clap". I got interrogated by the sargeant in the army and got angry—sex, guilt, and anger associated.

BOB

Birth description .... Breech, butt first, hospital birth. Mother out cold with anesthesia. I was the third of six children. My mother had three previous miscarriages. There was fear of loss or fear that I would die. At birth I had club feet. The OB team made fun and laughed at me.

How my birth affects my sexuality .... I have the fear I will hurt my partner. My partners reject me, proving there is something wrong with me. I am gay—I avoid hurting women. I do it differently than most men by being gay. I don't let myself get close and intimate to my partner out of lack of trust, and fear of hurting them, being hurt or being rejected. Sometimes I feel too guilty to have sex.

BHAKTI

Birth description . . . . Breech. I was twelve pounds when I was born. I hurt my mother. I was two weeks late. My mother was humiliated at my birth. She had two hundred and forty internal stitches. The oxygen was cut off through the umbilical cord.

How my birth affects my sexuality . . . . I'm too much, and I am too big for men. I like anal sex. I feel stifled by intimacy. I feel like my aliveness will hurt my partner. I hold back my sexual aliveness so I won't hurt my partner. I'm not good enough to have sex last. Sex in my relationships is only good for one year, then my relationships always go downhill. At one and a half years, my relationships always break up. This is because my sister was born when I was one and a half years old.

SHARON

Birth description . . . . I was a breech birth, I came out with the cord around my neck. During the last few weeks of my pregnancy, they thought I was dead.

How my birth affects my sexuality . . . . In sex, I feel I have no aliveness. I feel disassociated from my body. Sometimes I feel dead and unconscious in sex. I feel I have no choice of sexual partners—I feel like they have to choose me. I want to choose my own sexual partners now.

Face Presentation

GWENDOLYN

Birth description . . . . My parents wanted a boy. I came out face presentation. I got disapproval from the obstetrician, who was a friend of my father's. He said, "Another girl".

How my birth affects my sexuality . . . . I get a lot of disapproval from my mate about my femininity. My mates don't like to give me what I want. I like oral sex, and my partners never like to give that to me. I was not breastfed. I feel like I can't get what I want sexually, and I don't deserve to get what I want!

SANDY

Birth description .... I was a late birth. When I was ready to come, they held me back. My mother wanted a girl, and my father didn't want anything. I came out face presentation.

How my birth affects my sexuality .... I try to be asexual. I hide my sexuality. I put on a lot of weight so people can't see I am a woman.

CHRISTINA

Birth description .... I had my cord around my neck, and was face presentation. It was a long labor. My mother was asking, "What's wrong with my baby?" Heroin was administered in the first stage, gas and anesthesia in the second and third stages. I came down the birth canal facing the wrong way, and was physically turned by rocking movements. The cord was around my neck, and clamped as my head appeared. My father was home in bed all during my labor. He didn't visit until visiting hours, two hours later. I had no contact with my mother for thirteen hours after delivery. When I was delivered, I looked calm and doll-like.

How my birth affects my sexuality .... I feel that I am confused as to my sexuality—I wanted to be a boy. I have confusion about sensuality and femininity. Something is wrong with me; I am different from everyone else. I'm looking for someone just as different as I am for a partner. I fear relationships, therefore I have never entered into them, or had sex. I fear being controlled or smothered (suffocating in a relationship). I fear losing my power, becoming a subordinate.

Men aren't there for me—they don't support or understand me. I have a major feeling of fear of rejection. I fear that after sexual contact, they will withdraw, and not want me. That will prove that they only wanted me for their sexual gratification, not for love, caring and giving. Sex will take away my innocence unless it is within the confines of a committed relationship/marriage. I become unconscious, feel drugged and fearful, and have trouble breathing and moving energy when I become vulnerable sexually. But I look calm and in control and quiet, as if nothing is wrong.

Fast Birth

LINDA

Birth description .... My birth was quick and fast. My mother tore and had stiches.

How my birth affects my sexuality .... I feel my aliveness hurts my partner or myself. I feel out of control, and I fear really letting go in sex because I will hurt my partner. I hold back my sexual aliveness so no one gets hurts.

VIVIENNE

Birth description .... The birth was fast—only forty minutes of labor. My mother said she was ready, and the midwife said that was impossible. The male doctor never got there. I made the decision that I have to do it on my own without men.

How my birth affects my sexuality .... I am always looking for men to have sex with, and they are never there. I have a very healthy sexual appetite, and I feel guilty from my Catholic background. I get excited and want a man quickly, but men are not ready for me. I also like quick sex.

ROGER

Birth description .... I was born very fast. My Godmother delivered me. I was too fast, too soon.

How my birth affects my sexuality .... I want quick relationships and then I feel smothered. My first sexual experience was at eighteen and I was afraid to let go. I didn't have an orgasm. In sex, I am afraid to let go because I may be too much, or the experience may be too much.

ANITA

Birth description .... My mother told me that I came fast and that I was very beautiful. There were only women present at my birth.

How my birth affects my sexuality .... With men, I feel like I am in prison or a cell. I feel that I am wrong, and that women are worthless and don't deserve the men they want. I have attracted a lot of unavailable men with my beauty. I get into relationships quickly, and then I feel trapped and want to get out.

ANDERS

Birth description .... My mother was afraid at my birth—her mother had died at her birth. Mine was a quick birth and a disappointment because it was nothing special.

How my birth affects my sexuality .... I have guilt and fear of women's high expectations about sex. I feel there is nothing special about sex, and I have a fear of it. I also have a fear that my partner will be disappointed because the sexual experience will be nothing special for her.

NORMAN

Birth description .... The birth happened quickly.

How my birth affects my sexuality .... I feel wanted by my partner, but my sex life feels insufficient and repressed. I reach orgasm quickly, and women are not ready and excited. My ejaculation is premature and I feel insufficient.

LIDDY

Birth description .... A fast birth. I was a big baby. I hurt my mother. I was anesthetized. My father was not there. My father wanted a boy.

How my birth affects my sexuality .... I feel not good enough as a woman. I am too much for most men. Men are not there for me. It's easy for me to be attracted to someone and feel sexual energy, but then I make myself wrong for having sexual energy. In the past, I went unconscious except when I felt totally safe and appreciated by my partner. Men run away from me. I make myself wrong and guilty for putting out sexual energy, yes/no energy. I am afraid of intimacy—wild sex is safer because I don't feel vulnerable. I have a fear of being hurt. I am guilty about being a sexual being. I feel guilty about putting out sexual energy and enjoying it. I don't allow myself total pleasure.

I create disasters to avoid relationships. When I go for a relationship 100%, I make myself wrong. I'm like a see-saw.

Held Back

KAL

Birth description . . . . My mother held me back at my birth.

How my birth affects my sexuality . . . . I don't trust men. I am afraid to show by body because no one will want me or love me. I feel I am not enough or sufficient. I have to be always strong. If I am vulnerable in sex, then I feel not strong and sufficient. I felt I was not in control at my birth because I couldn't come when I wanted to. I try to stay in control in sex.

LARS ERIC

Birth description . . . . My mother was left alone, and she had a fear no one would be there when I was born. I felt that I was coming too fast. My mother held me back out of fear of being alone when I was born.

How my birth affects my sexuality . . . . Women hold me back out of their fear of sex. I am extremely tentative about sex because I don't want to make women afraid. I have the thought that I am not good enough and this affects me sexually. I get held back by women if I come on too fast sexually.

ELLEN

Birth description . . . . I was held back at my birth.

How my birth affects my sexuality . . . . I feel held back in sex. I won't say what I want. I won't say I want "it", or ask for "it". I haven't had sex in the last year of my marriage.

DONNA

Birth description . . . . I was held back to wait for the doctor. My birth was controlled, and I had to wait for men. After I was held back, then they pulled me out with forceps.

How my birth affects my sexuality . . . . I am still waiting for a man to be available to me. I choose men who are married or live in other cities or countries. I rebelled against control and structure, I like sex best when it is forbidden, wild and a mystery. I don't belong here, everyone comes before I do, especially men. The men I want never want me 100%.

Dry Birth

VERA

Birth description . . . . My birth was a dry birth. The waters broke twenty-four hours before I was born.

How my birth affects my sexuality . . . . I can't get anything. I have the thought I can't do it, and I have a lot of irritation about sex. I can't have enough sex. I want to get pregnant and I can't do that either. I have a lot of frustration around sex because my conditioning is that sex is for babies. I can't make babies, so sex brings up guilt and irritation like my mother had at my birth.

Induced

FAITH

Birth description . . . . The doctor threatened to induce me if I wasn't born on the day I was born.

How my birth affects my sexuality . . . . I liked to be seduced into sex with music and a massage.

CHRISTOPHER

Birth description . . . . My father wanted me to be born on his birthday. He had my mother run a lot so the baby would come on his birthday. I was born on his birthday.

How my birth affects my sexuality . . . . I strongly identify with my father. I have a thin, underdeveloped body like his. My father was also a priest who married. I was twenty-four before I made love to a women. I did it out of a feeling of desperation, that something must be wrong with me if I hadn't had sex by that time. I pretended to have sex the first time. Her parents were in the house and I masturbated her. I finally made love to her when I was drunk.

I masturbate a lot. I feel deep shame when I masturbate. I feel deeply embarrassed by my sexuality. I was told that God and my parents would love me more if I didn't have sex. I always have to be induced into sex by my partner.

DIANE

Birth description . . . . I was induced and heavily anesthetized at my birth.

How my birth affects my sexuality . . . . I always feel like I am in a fog sexually. I resent being manipulated and controlled by my partner. I always have to wait for my partner to initiate sex, so then I can feel manipulated and get angry like I did at my birth.

DUNCAN

Birth description . . . . Induced, drugs, forceps. I wasn't ready to come. I was late.

How my birth affects my sexuality . . . . Feel manipulated and controlled by women. Women have to initiate sex. Go unconscious during sex. Go unconscious around having sex. I'm not there for my partner when she wants me sexually.

JACQUE

Birth description . . . . Forceps/induced. I was a ten-month baby who didn't want to come out because my mother was afraid my father would be angry when he found out I was a girl. I was induced, but my mother was told she would probably need a C-section. However, I was born in two hours. My mom remembers two contractions and then she was anesthetized. I was pulled out by forceps when I felt like I was doing it just fine on my own. My head was deformed, and needed massage and re-positioning for a month. When I was brought to my parents after delivery, they sent me back to the nursery, not believing I was their child because of my head. So I thought, "There is something wrong with me."

How my birth affects my sexuality .... I sometimes feel I'm being "pushed" to come in a hurry. I had the thought "I am sexually undesirable". So I created men rejecting me sexually. I have had the thought I was fat (my mom's small pelvis). I have had the fear that another woman would seduce my mate because there was something wrong with me sexually. I have had the thought that it isn't safe to come out sexually. What has healed me and helped me let go sexually is doing the "Sexuality Sexercises". I felt very stuck in my sex case until I started scheduling sex and doing the book at the same time.

Late Birth

MARY

Birth description .... I was born too late; I need lots of time.

How my birth affects my sexuality .... I don't like to reveal myself to men because I feel not good enough. I feel that I am too much. Men always have to wait for me. I have put on weight to keep men away.

JONAS

Birth description .... I was one week late. My mother was afraid to let me out. I had the thought at my birth that there was something wrong with me.

How my birth affects my sexuality .... I have to always wait for sex from women, then I come quickly. I feel that there is something wrong with me sexually as a man.

ROLF

Birth description .... I did not want to come out at my birth. I was two weeks late. I was the third boy. I didn't want to come as a boy.

How my birth affects my sexuality .... I have partners who do not want me as a man. I hold back my sexuality because I feel unwanted as a man. I have fear and guilt about sex. I also have fear of being close and vulnerable.

PAM

Birth description .... I was three weeks late. They turned me in the womb. My mother said I almost killed her, I came out so fast. I was anesthetized. I felt comfortable in the womb—I didn't want to come out. My mom was uncomfortable.

How my birth affects my sexuality .... I like to do things my way. I am rebellious. My space and comfort are important to me. I resist doing things when others want me to. I have sex and do things on my own time. I am dangerous, I hurt people I love. I keep separate to avoid hurting people I love. I sabotage relationships.

I was in a relationship with another woman. I liked to manipulate the relationship and my partner. We got in a very bad car accident when I was driving and fell asleep at the wheel. My partner was almost killed, and I was hurt very badly. We were taken to separate hospitals. There was a lot of guilt on my part for causing pain and hurt to my partner, just like I felt I had hurt my mother. The accident re-created my birth, as both situations had unconsciousness and the result of almost killing the one I loved as well as myself.

Caesarean

SARA

Birth description .... I was a planned caesarean, and during the surgery, my mother was sterilized. I had no bonding with my mother because she was sick for six weeks after the surgery. I had bottled breast milk.

How my birth affects my sexuality .... I have the thought that no one is there for me. The first time I had sex, I didn't know I was supposed to enjoy it. I had the conditioning that nice girls don't, and that sex is only for when you are married. I always feel naughty when I have sex. I am also attracted to men that are not there for me. Most of the men I am attracted to are unavailable and usually married.

SHARON

Birth description .... I was a planned caesarean. A boy baby had died before I was born, so they planned the caesarean so I would live. There was a lot of fear that I would die. I had the fear that I could kill someone with my aliveness. My mother and I were very drugged at the birth.

How my birth affects my sexuality . . . . I hold back my aliveness out of fear of hurting my partner. I have a lot of guilt when I enjoy sex. In my early days with sex, I often would be drugged or passed out like at my birth. Sometimes, after sex, I wondered what had happened to me, like I must have thought about being born caesarean.

RACHEL

Birth description . . . . I was a caesarean. I was taken away from my mother and put in an incubator. I felt very separate—I had no bonding with my mother.

How my birth affects my sexuality . . . . I feel separate from my partners. I feel disconnected from the experience of sex. I have a tendency to want men I can't have.

GUNNELL

Birth description . . . . I was supposed to be a boy. My mother had a still-born before me, so there was fear that something would happen to me. I was a planned caesarean. I was three weeks early.

How my birth affects my sexuality . . . . I have always suppressed my sexuality, and I feel unwanted by men. I feel that sex is either disgusting, or if it is good, I am abandoned by the man. Sometimes I need a lot of time in sex. Sometimes sex is very fast, with lots of drugs. I drink a lot of coffee, which feels like a drug to me. I feel that I haven't come out sexually yet.

LISA

Birth description . . . . I was a planned caesarean with a boy's named picked out. My mother's stomach was moving up and down. I was really moving around. When the doctor opened my mother's stomach, he said, "You were already screaming." I was separated and put in an incubator.

How my birth affects my sexuality . . . . My thought is that I was angry at having my birth controlled, and that I couldn't do it my way. I act this out by having a lot of anger at men, and by feeling controlled by men and women. I like to do things my own way. Also, as a result of my birth, I love to find shortcuts and I always say, "I am taking the path of least resistance." I often do things easily and without struggle, including getting three promotions in three months, and skipping a lot of rungs on the corporate ladder.

I avoid relationships by excelling in my career. I have had very few relationships with men that were long term. I had two relationships that lasted one year each. My separation issue has kept me from getting close to people. I have the thought that people will not want me if they get close to me. They will reject me. In sex, I want to remain in control. I don't have orgasms unless I do it myself.

SUZANNE

Birth description . . . . I was caesarean and drugged. They wanted a boy, and they put me in an incubator.

How my birth affects my sexuality . . . . I like to be "high" in sex. I have created partners who use drugs to be high, which keeps them separate from me. I like to get sex over quickly. I have a hard time being held, and I can't face my partner after sex.

Birth Case Histories—Birth Situations

The Baby Was Hurt at Birth, or there Was Something Wrong with the Baby

TOM

Birth description . . . . My parents were nervous about my birth. My brother's birth had been difficult. I was born at home. The doctor was in a hurry because he had to go to another birth. When I came out, the thought was that there was something wrong with me.

How my birth affects my sexuality . . . . I hurry to make women want me. I always have to prove that I am OK as a man sexually.

MONICA

Birth description . . . . I was born in Europe, during the war, in the middle of an air raid. My birth was "hurry up or die." My father was not there—he was at war. I had swollen breasts at my birth and the doctor said, "Look at this hot number." He cut my nipples to release the pressure of them being swollen.

How my birth affects my sexuality . . . . Men are not there for me sexually. Also, I feel men will hurt me, and that they don't respect me. My sex life is like an air raid: short lived and intense.

MARK

Birth description . . . . I had a broken collarbone at my birth. The thought was that there was something wrong with me.

How my birth affects my sexuality . . . . I hold myself back sexually so I won't be hurt.

JANEY

Birth description . . . . I should not have been there, I was unplanned. My mother took anti-malaria pills—there were spasms in the womb. I felt my mother trying to get rid of me. I was born very fast. The doctor didn't get there in time. Mother was drugged after the birth, and I felt abandoned. I had to hold back my aliveness for my mother's sake because she was hysterical. I have a hearing problem which is from my mother taking the anti-malaria pills when I was in the womb.

How my birth affects my sexuality . . . . I never think that the man I want, wants me. If he does want me, I don't want him. Also, I always think there is something wrong with me or my relationship.

CHRISTINA

Birth description . . . . My parents had a fear that there would be something wrong with me because there were a lot of handicapped or dumb children in the family. I felt that I had to be good in the womb, so my mother would know I was all right. At my birth, my mother was scared and my father was not there. My mother was also afraid of the midwife, who was not very nice.

How my birth affects my sexuality . . . . To be a women is to be scared. I can't surrender sexually because of my fear. I also fear that there is something wrong with me sexually.

RUNER

Birth description . . . . My midwife hurt me at my birth.

How my birth affects my sexuality . . . . I feel guilty that I have confused feelings about sex. I feel rejected by women. I feel women hurt me sexually, and I always fear being hurt by a woman. I fear surrendering to a woman. I feel that I am not good enough to have what I want, and I feel I don't fit in.

KATHERINE

Birth description . . . . They wanted a girl because boy babies died. My first brother died two days after he was born. He was a blue baby. There were several miscarriages before me. There was a fear that I would not make it. They thought that if I did make it, there might be something wrong with me. After I was born, they carried me around on a pillow like I was a fragile princess.

How my birth affects my sexuality . . . . I feel that anything that goes wrong sexually is my fault. I'm not good enough to keep my partner sexually satisfied—there is something wrong with me. I feel guilty that all the boys in the family died. My younger brother died also, and so did my father. Men don't live that I am close to.

While I was in a homosexual relationship, coming from my male energy, I went over a freeway embankment and had extensive injuries and broken bones. It was a miracle that I made it through the accident alive, and was later able to walk without limping or permanent damage. I really went through the thought that the men in my family, or the masculine energy, dies. After going through a period of sexual confusion, I am now dating men again and back loving my feminine self.

JACKIE

Birth description . . . . My mother wanted a boy. My father didn't care about having children. I was two weeks late. I was anesthetized at my birth. The obstetrician broke my foot when I came out.

How my birth affects my sexuality . . . . I denied my femininity by getting heavy and having male-oriented jobs. Men hurt me. There is something wrong with me, especially sexually. Men disapprove of me in everything, but especially sexually.

SANDY

Birth description .... I felt there was something wrong with me because I wasn't a boy. I felt rejection and separation at my birth. When I was born, they said I had big shoulders and a big head. They said I looked like a boy.

How my birth affects my sexuality .... In my relationships, my partners focus on my body instead of what I am on the inside. I have gotten big and heavy to keep men away and affirm that there is something wrong with me. It's safer to keep men away because I fear separation, abandonment and abuse by men.

The Baby Was the Wrong Sex

ELLIE

Birth description .... I was the last planned child of five girls. My parents wanted a boy. They were disappointed at my birth because I was a girl.

How my birth affects my sexuality .... Sex is often a disappointment. I feel I have to accommodate men. "Girls don't matter" is the message I received as I was growing up. My father always preached that sex is dirty, sex is only for having children, not for excitement. I don't trust men and I feel men don't want me. If a man wants me, I hold back. I don't really believe they want me as a woman or sexually.

ENRIQUE

Birth description .... I was wanted but they wanted a boy. When I was born, my father was extremely disappointed that I was not a boy.

How my birth affects my sexuality .... I want sex, but I am afraid of sex at the same time. I think my body is ugly and a disappointment. Sooner or later, men always leave me. I have to struggle to get a man's love. I cannot enjoy sex because I struggle too much to keep the man pleased. I don't want my partner to be disappointed in me.

The Mother Was Hurt at the Birth

MATILDA

Birth description .... I was guilty at birth about hurting my mother.

How my birth affects my sexuality .... I have pain and violence hooked up with sex.

MAUDE

Birth description .... My father did not want me. I hurt my mother at my birth. My father was not at my birth.

How my birth affects my sexuality .... Men are not there for me and they leave me. I had incest with both my father and my uncle. I feel I hurt women by having sex with their husbands. I feel safer alone, without men. Then no one gets hurt. I live five hundred miles away from my partner.

JORGEN

Birth description .... I hurt my mother at my birth.

How my birth affects my sexuality .... I get sex over quickly. I hold back my aliveness so I won't hurt my partner.

ARNE

Birth description .... My mother had thirty-eight hours of labor and she felt like she was dying. I feel I hurt my mother.

How my birth affects my sexuality .... I feel I don't deserve pleasure. I feel guilty about hurting my mother, and I have orgasms and hurt connected.

MISHA

Birth description .... At birth I started coming out and this created problems because the doctor wasn't there, and they thought that I was too early. I felt like I hurt my mother and I was separate.

How my birth affects my sexuality . . . . I feel I hurt my husband and daughters when I left the relationship. I wasn't satisfied sexually. That was one of the main reasons I left—to have what I want sexually. What I want sexually hurts people I love.

ANDERS

Birth description . . . . My mother wanted a girl. I felt that I hurt my mother at birth.

How my birth affects my sexuality . . . . I choose women who are used to being abused. I feel that pain follows pleasure. Around sex, I feel evil and guilty. I have confusion around sex: I see the holy side and the sinful side. My confusion around sex makes me feel split, and like I am a victim of sex.

MATHEW

Birth description . . . . At my birth I was vulnerable and I was handled roughly. I feel that I hurt my mother. I was also angry. I was separated from my mother for quite a while after birth, and I was breast-fed on schedule.

How my birth affects my sexuality . . . . I have the fear I will hurt women in sex, so I hold back my aliveness sexually. It is easier for me to fantasize about sex than to have sex. I don't feel safe to have an orgasm inside a woman. In my last relationship, I felt held back sexually. We would start and stop.

I have so much guilt about sex. I think it is tied up with hurting my mother. I feel that I will hurt women if I leave. I feel that you are supposed to be married to have sex. I got married to a woman soon after I had sex with her because I was guilty. The relationship didn't work, so it is hard for me now just to have sex for pleasure. I always feel separate from my partner after orgasm. It is not safe to be vulnerable in an intimate relationship. I have the thoughts I can't get what I want. I can't ask for what I want and I don't know what I want.

The Father Was Not Present at the Birth

EVA

Birth description . . . . My father was not at my birth.

How my birth affects my sexuality . . . . Men are not there for me when I need them or want them, especially sexually. "I can't get enough sex" is another thought I have. I have created being physically abused by the men that I have had intimate sexual relationships with.

JUSTINE

Birth description . . . . My birth was OK, but my father had to leave. He wasn't there for me.

How my birth affects my sexuality . . . . Men say that they want me and then they don't act like they want me. I feel that I hurt men to get even with my father.

MARRIANNE

Birth description . . . . I was heavily drugged at my birth. I was conceived by my mother to keep my father in the marriage. When I was born, my father didn't come to the birth, and he never came back. He was having a deep relationship with another woman. They took care of my mother more than me at birth.

How my birth affects my sexuality . . . . I feel that men can't really love me. I am not loved as a woman. I created incest situations where the man is not there for me. I create men that are always in relationships with other women. I have pain and sadness hooked up with sex because men always leave me. I feel that in sex I work hard to please the man, more than myself. I took care of my mother more than I was taken care of. In sex, it is important for me to have cuddling and closeness to make up for the bonding I didn't have at birth. I have used drugs in the past when having sex in order to feel more.

BRITT

Birth description . . . . My father wanted a boy. He was not at my birth because he got a cold that day.

How my birth affects my sexuality . . . . Men are not there for me when I need them. I can't ask for what I want sexually, and I can't get what I want sexually from a man.

The Baby Had a Long Separation from Its Mother

LEIF

Birth description . . . . My midwife was a harsh woman with no feelings. I was separated from my mother for twenty-four hours.

How my birth affects my sexuality . . . . I feel very separate from women, and women don't want me. I have the thoughts "I can't have sex the way I want it", and "Women will reject me sexually".

CAROLINE

Birth description . . . . I was taken away from my mother at birth for a day. My father was in another city the day I was born.

How my birth affects my sexuality . . . . I don't feel good enough to enjoy sex fully. My husband and I are always going through separations. I feel separate from the ones I love.

The Baby Was Stuck

MONA

Birth description . . . . I was stuck at my birth.

How my birth affects my sexuality . . . . I feel stuck in relationships, and I want to get out. I feel guilty about sex. Feeling guilty about sex makes me feel stuck about sex.

JODIE

Birth description . . . . I was wanted as a little girl. I was stuck at my birth and couldn't get out. I felt like I was doing it alone, and with a lot of struggle.

How my birth affects my sexuality . . . . I feel stuck in being a little girl. My father left as I matured. I have the thought that men will leave me if I am mature. I am angry and frustrated with men. I got a breast implant to be more of a woman. The more sexy and like a woman I feel, the more alone I feel.

PHYLISS

Birth description . . . . I was stuck in the birth canal. My mother said as I was coming out, "I don't care if she dies, just get her out of here."

How my birth affects my sexuality . . . . I feel stuck and entrapped when having sex. When sex is really good, I feel trapped. I am afraid of having sex be really great, because I might die then.

The Baby Was Adopted at Birth

VERA

Birth description . . . . I was supposed to be adopted at birth. I felt alone. I was not adopted until I was two months old.

How my birth affects my sexuality . . . . I feel unwanted and unloved. I always attract the wrong men. I attract men who do not want me sexually.

There Was Almost a Miscarriage

SYLVIA

Birth description . . . . They almost lost me—there was almost a miscarriage. My mother was bleeding in the hospital. I had the thought that everything I do is a problem for my mother. My father died.

How my birth affects my sexuality . . . . Normal men leave me. The man I love leaves me. I might as well not have sex because men leave me anyway. I always have to struggle to get love and sex, just the way I had to struggle to live.

The Mother Tried to Abort the Baby

ANNETTE

Birth description .... My mother was sad, confused and angry about being pregnant. My father did not want me or my mother. My mother tried to abort me because she was afraid to have a child on her own.

How my birth affects my sexuality .... I always think men don't want me. I always feel stuck and irritable about having sex and relationships. I always have to struggle to find a sexual partner, and to have sex with a man who wants me.

YVONNE

Birth description .... I was unwanted, and my mother attempted to abort me.

How my birth affects my sexuality .... I have a need to be wanted as a woman. At birth I struggled, and now I struggle to be wanted sexually, and to be good enough as a woman.

The Baby Was Circumcised Right After Birth

JOEL

Birth description .... I was separated from my mother and circumcised right after birth.

How my birth affects my sexuality .... I have the attitude that I can't trust anyone. I especially can't trust being touched.

PATRICK

Birth description .... My mother and I were drugged at my birth, and then they pulled me out with forceps. I was put in an incubator and circumcised within the first hour and a half after my birth.

How my birth affects my sexuality . . . . I feel I can't trust anyone about sexuality and vulnerability. I weighed four hundred pounds at one time. I used my weight to protect myself and stay separate.

Struggle at Birth

DAVID

Birth description . . . . At my birth, there was lots of struggle with my mother. My mother was angry at me already, maybe from some past life struggles we had together.

How my birth affects my sexuality . . . . My sexual relationships in the past have been such a struggle that I avoid them completely now. I always choose women who don't want me. If a woman wants me, it is too uncomfortable and unfamiliar, so I make excuses to leave the relationship. I am a good giver in sex, but I don't trust women enough to receive from them. I always choose unavailable women, and mostly long distance relationships. I am a workaholic. I use work to avoid relationships. I am unwanted by women, and it is safer to be alone.

Our Personal Lie and How to Discover It

Our Personal Lie is our most negative thought about ourselves. This lie was a decision we made about ourselves based on a reaction we had to something our parents felt or said about us.

We could have decided what our Personal Lie was at conception. If our parents did not want us, or we were illegitimate, our Personal Lie would be either I AM UNWANTED, or I AM ILLEGITIMATE. The Personal Lie could be a decision we made in the womb. If our parents were worried about money, we could decide I AM A FINANCIAL BURDEN. If there was a fear that something might be wrong with the baby due to an attempted abortion or a previous problem with another child, the Personal Lie could be THERE IS SOMETHING WRONG WITH ME. If we felt we hurt our mother at birth because she was in pain, cut, or anesthetized, the Personal Lie could be I HURT PEOPLE or I AM GUILTY FOR THE PAIN I CAUSED MY MOTHER. If someone at our birth said "what an ugly baby", we could decide I AM UGLY.

I chose my Personal Lie at my birth. For seven seconds, my father was disappointed that I was a girl, so I decided I was a disappointment as a woman/girl. My Personal Lie is I AM A DISAPPOINTMENT AS A WOMAN.

We make the Personal Lie real in our life. After the seven seconds, my father was thrilled with me, happy I was healthy, and really loved me. He forgot his initial reaction to me, but I held on to it, and beat myself up with it for thirty-five years.

I expected to be a disappointment to all men who loved me just like I had been a disappointment to my father. If men were not disappointed in me, I would make sure to do something to disappoint them in order to keep proving this thought. I also was disappointed by men.

We either indulge in our Personal Lie by acting it out, creating people being disappointed in us, not wanting us, etc . . . or we overcompensate for our Personal Lie by bending over backwards to prove that we are really wanted, good enough, or a wonderful surprise.

Often people use their Personal Lie to develop their careers. They are overcompensating for the negative thought by choosing a career that proves the opposite. For example, a doctor, healer, chiropracter, or rebirther could have the Personal Lie I HURT PEOPLE. A person who has the thought I AM UGLY could be a model make-up artist or beautician. A person with the thought I AM GUILTY could be a lawyer, always working to prove his client's innocence. An actor could have the Personal Lie NO ONE NOTICES ME or I'M NOT GOOD ENOUGH.

Each person has to analyze their own mind, and see what thought motivates their whole life. For example, my Personal Lie is that I AM A DISAPPOINTMENT AS A WOMAN. Other women with similar stories of being the wrong sex could have the thought I AM UNWANTED AS A WOMAN, or I AM NOT GOOD ENOUGH AS A WOMAN or I AM WRONG AS A WOMAN, or I AM THE OPPOSITE OF WHAT PEOPLE EXPECT AS A WOMAN. I have thought all these things at times. The thought that has the most charge is usually the right one. If someone has a real right/wrong issue, and is always trying to prove they are right, the thought I AM WRONG AS A WOMAN will probably have the most charge.

Discovering your Personal Lie is very valuable because we beat ourselves up with this thought in our careers, our sex lives, with our money, our bodies, and basically in our relationships with everyone and everything. By locating the thought, we can see it as a lie, laugh at it, decide to be wrong about it, and choose another thought or decision called an Eternal Law. Our Eternal Law is our highest thought about ourselves. We take our Personal Lie and change it into a positive affirmation. For example, my Personal Lie, I AM

A DISAPPOINTMENT AS A WOMAN, becomes my Eternal Law, I AM A SURPRISINGLY WONDERFUL WOMAN.

If your Personal Lie is I AM UNWANTED, the Eternal Law is I AM WANTED, or I AM WANTED AS A MAN, or I AM WANTED AS A WOMAN. The Personal Lie, I AM GUILTY, becomes the Eternal Law, I AM INNOCENT. The Personal Lie, THERE IS SOMETHING WRONG WITH ME, becomes the Eternal Law, I AM PERFECT JUST AS I AM. The Personal Lie, I HURT PEOPLE, becomes the Eternal Law, I BENEFIT, HEAL, AND PLEASURE PEOPLE WITH MY ALIVENESS. The Personal Lie, I AM NOT GOOD ENOUGH, becomes the Eternal Law, I AM GOOD ENOUGH. The Personal Lie, I AM UGLY, becomes the Eternal Law, I AM BEAUTIFUL.

Sometimes it is difficult to locate your Personal Lie because of other thoughts blocking you from finding the most negative thought. For instance, at first I thought my Personal Lie was I AM CONFUSED, because I was confused about my sexuality. Often when people have the thought "I can't", they feel they can't find their Personal Lie. "I can't" comes from helplessness, and it is often related to feeling helpless and like a victim at birth. Often people have to change the "I can't" thought to "I can", before they can find their deeper-level Personal Lie. Until they are willing to see that they can, they can't find their Personal Lie.

"I don't know" is another thought that blocks people from finding their Personal Lie. This thought also comes from helplessness, and must be changed to "I know everything", so that the Personal Lie can be discovered. For many people, "I can't" or "I don't know" could be their first Personal Lie, until they move through those decisions about life.

Some people have the Personal Lie, I DO NOT WANT TO BE THERE, or I AM NOT SUPPOSED TO BE HERE, if their parents tried to abort them or they did not like life from the beginning. People who are born with their cords around their necks often are trying to commit suicide in the womb. Their thought could be either, I DON'T WANT TO BE THERE or I AM NOT SUPPOSED TO BE HERE.

Sometimes when you are trying to discover your Personal Lie, you might get in touch with a result of your Personal Lie instead, such as I AM NOT SMART ENOUGH, I AM NOT THIN ENOUGH, I AM NOT PRETTY ENOUGH, I AM NOT SEXY ENOUGH, I AM NOT SUCCESSFUL ENOUGH, I AM NOT TALL ENOUGH.

All these balloons are negative thoughts we could have about ourselves, but they are really a result of the Personal Lie, I AM NOT GOOD ENOUGH. If the Personal Lie, I AM NOT GOOD ENOUGH, is erased or released, all the helium balloons such as I am NOT SMART ENOUGH, PRETTY

ENOUGH, THIN ENOUGH, SEXY ENOUGH, SUCCESSFUL ENOUGH, TALL ENOUGH, will fly off and leave. The bottom line negative thought is I AM NOT GOOD ENOUGH. When the Eternal Law, I AM GOOD ENOUGH, is integrated into the body, then all the other thoughts are healed. The reality becomes BECAUSE I AM GOOD ENOUGH, I AM SMART ENOUGH, I AM THIN ENOUGH, I AM PRETTY ENOUGH, I AM SEXY ENOUGH, I AM SUCCESSFUL ENOUGH, and I AM TALL ENOUGH.

To locate your Personal Lie, fill in the blanks in the following statements.

1. My most negative thought about myself is that
   I am ________.

2. What I am most afraid people will find out about me is that
   I am ________.

3. The reason I can't have what I want is that I am ________.

4. The reason I don't deserve what I want is that I am ________.

5. My most negative thought about myself is that I am ________.

Now choose the thought that comes up the most often. If all of the thoughts are different, choose the one that gives you the most charge in your body. In other words, the one you like the least. Once you find your Personal Lie, for example, I AM NOT GOOD ENOUGH, change the thought to your Eternal Law, I AM GOOD ENOUGH. if you have the Personal Lie, I AM NOT GOOD ENOUGH, you might feel that the thought, I AM NOT GOOD ENOUGH, is not good enough to be your Personal Lie. If you have the Personal Lie, I AM NOT WANTED, you will not want that thought. If you have the Personal Lie, I AM WRONG, you will try to make your Personal Lie wrong.

Use your intuition to find the right thought. Once you discover your Personal Lie, change the thought to your Eternal Law. Put your Eternal Law on index cards and put them up all over the house: on the refrigerator, the bathroom mirror, in your car, etc., to remind yourself of the truth about yourself, the Eternal Law. The Eternal Law will feel like a lie until you integrate it into your body. Notice your resistance to changing your Personal Lie to your Eternal Law. We cling to our negative decisions, because we are used to them and have adapted to them. By constantly seeing your Eternal Law plastered all over your car, house and work environment, you will start to believe it. I also suggest that you write your Eternal Law twenty times a day for one month, with a response column.

ETERNAL LAW	**RESPONSE**
I am good enough.	Not really.

Once you no longer have any negative responses, you are starting to integrate the thought. Write it for at least one more week after that. You have lived with your Personal Lie all your life. This thought has motivated you to overcompensate for it, or to indulge in it. This thought is your survival. You have survived all your life with this thought, and it will often hang on. It is important to really affirm your Eternal Law until you integrate it, and feel it in your body. It is not enough just to accept your Eternal Law intellectually. It goes much deeper than that. You have to accept it in every one of your cells. Once you have really accepted this thought, all aspects of your life will really change.

We are really addicted to our Personal Lies just as we are addicted to drugs, alcohol, food etc. We have to get off the addiction to our Personal Lies just as we would get off a food, alcohol, or drug addiction. We have to admit to the addiction, and say, "no" to it. Since we have survived with this Personal Lie, we fear giving it up. Even if our lives don't work because of these thoughts, we are used to them, and are more afraid of change, and having something worse happen, than we are of keeping these sabotaging thoughts.

If a person has the Personal Lie, I AM UNWANTED, they are addicted to being unwanted. It is safe, familiar and comfortable to be unwanted. They will choose people who don't want them as intimate partners. They will chase after these people who don't want them. If the person then wants them, they will run away because they only feel safe being unwanted. They have to learn to surrender to being wanted. They have to really believe the Eternal Law that they are wanted.

Often to help make the change from our Personal Lie to our Eternal Law, we have to write a few other affirmations at the same time. Affirmations such as IT'S SAFE TO CHANGE, MY LIFE IS INEVITABLE, and I AM WANTED. By writing these three thoughts for one month, you would gain a whole new experience of your aliveness and who you are. You would feel happier, more alive and excited about life.

A Course in Miracles explains that your ego is the collection of negative thoughts you have about yourself, which doesn't want you to change. Sometimes locating your Personal Lie can be tricky because your ego likes you to stay stuck in it. If you have trouble finding or releasing your Personal Lie, see a rebirther, and or take the Loving Relationships Training. (Check Appendix B for information about the Loving Relationships Training and LRT-sponsored rebirthers.) The Loving Relationships Training, in the basic LRT weekend, does extensive work to locate and start to release the Personal Lie.

Our Personal Lie and Its Correlation to Our Biggest Problem With Sex

What I have noticed over the last three years of doing research on sexuality, is that our Personal Lie is directly related to our biggest problem with sex. Actually, our biggest problem with sex is a direct result of our Personal Lie. If we clear our Personal Lie, we are able to have cosmic, orgasmic, blissful sex.

This chapter includes people's Personal Lies and their biggest problems with sex. Included with each person's Personal Lie and biggest problem with sex is their Sexual Eternal Law.

The examples given below are the thoughts of people from around the world. These people were participants in sexuality courses in England, Sweden, Australia, New Zealand, Florida, California, Georgia and Alaska. In the European trainings, there were people from Germany, France, Denmark, Finland, and Ireland. The thoughts are organized according to the Personal Lies. In subsequent chapters, there are longer sexual histories which explain in more detail many people's Personal Lies and how they affect their sex lives.

KEY TO ABBREVIATIONS

PL = Personal Lie

PS = Biggest Problem With Sex

SEL = Sexual Eternal Law

PL: I Am Not Good Enough.

PS: I don't reach a state of ecstasy.
SEL: I AM GOOD ENOUGH TO REACH A STATE OF ECSTASY.

PS: I can't please myself or my partner.
SEL: I AM GOOD ENOUGH TO PLEASE MYSELF AND MY PARTNER SEXUALLY.

PS: I don't reach orgasm.
SEL: I AM GOOD ENOUGH TO REACH ORGASM.

PS: I can't let go and relax.

SEL: I AM GOOD ENOUGH TO LET GO AND RELAX.

PS: No one wants all that I have to give.
SEL: I AM GOOD ENOUGH TO HAVE A SEXUAL PARTNER WHO WANTS ALL THAT I HAVE TO GIVE.

PS: I worry that I am not good enough sexually.
SEL: I AM GOOD ENOUGH TO BE SEXUALLY GOOD ENOUGH.

PS: I attract women whom I can't satisfy sexually.
SEL: I AM GOOD ENOUGH TO SEXUALLY SATISFY THE WOMAN I LOVE.

PS: I can't get close enough to have a good time. I'm scared of letting go.
SEL: I'M GOOD ENOUGH TO GET CLOSE ENOUGH TO HAVE A GOOD TIME IN SEX. IT'S SAFE TO LET GO.

PS: I'm not good enough to live up to my partner's high expectations about sex.
SEL: I'M GOOD ENOUGH TO LIVE UP TO MY PARTNER'S HIGH EXPECTATIONS ABOUT SEX.

PS: Sex makes me exhausted.
SEL: I AM GOOD ENOUGH TO HAVE SEX EXHILARATE AND PLEASURE ME.

PS: I am afraid of sexual energy.
SEL: I AM GOOD ENOUGH TO ENJOY AND BE PLEASURED BY SEXUAL ENERGY.

PS: Sex starts out great, and then declines.
SEL: I'M GOOD ENOUGH TO KEEP SEX EXCITING, GREAT AND PLEASURABLE.

PS: I can't initiate sex.
SEL: I'M GOOD ENOUGH TO INITIATE SEX, PLEASURE MY PARTNER, AND BE PLEASURED.

PS: Sex is good in the beginning and then turns bad. I can't ask for what I want.

SEL: I'M GOOD ENOUGH TO SUSTAIN GREAT SEX ALWAYS WITH MY PARTNER, AND TO ASK FOR AND RECEIVE WHAT I WANT SEXUALLY.

PS: I avoid sex—it's too much trouble and overwhelms me.
SEL: I'M GOOD ENOUGH TO HAVE SEX WITH THE MAN (WOMAN) I WANT, THE WAY I WANT IT, EASILY AND EFFORTLESSLY.

PS: I don't have enough sex: I don't want my wife sexually.
SEL: SINCE I KNOW I AM GOOD ENOUGH, I HAVE ENOUGH SEX, AND I REALLY WANT MY WIFE SEXUALLY.

PS: If I have too much pleasure, I will disappear.
SEL: SINCE I KNOW I AM GOOD ENOUGH, THE MORE PLEASURE I EXPERIENCE, THE SAFER AND MORE POWERFUL I FEEL.

PL: I Am Unwanted.

PS: I don't want sex with my husband.
SEL: SINCE I KNOW I AM WANTED, I WANT SEX WITH THE MAN WHO WANTS ME, MY HUSBAND.

PS: I can't get sex when I want it.
SEL: SINCE I KNOW I AM WANTED, I CAN HAVE SEX WHENEVER I WANT.

PS: I will be sent away if I have sex.
SEL: SINCE I KNOW I AM WANTED, PEOPLE WANT ME TO STAY WHEN I HAVE GREAT SEX.

PS: My partner has premature ejaculations.
SEL: SINCE I KNOW I AM WANTED, MY PARTNER WANTS ME ENOUGH TO GIVE AND RECEIVE SEXUAL PLEASURE WITH ME FOR AS LONG AS I WANT.

PS: My partner is not interested in having sex with me.
SEL: SINCE I KNOW I AM WANTED, MY PARTNER REALLY WANTS ME SEXUALLY.

PS: I can't find a partner for sex.

SEL: SINCE I KNOW I AM WANTED, IT'S EASY TO FIND A PARTNER I WANT FOR SEX.

PS: Sex is unavailable.
SEL: SINCE I KNOW I AM WANTED, SEX IS ALWAYS AVAILABLE TO ME WHEN I WANT IT.

PS: It's not safe to surrender in sex.
SEL: SINCE I KNOW I AM WANTED, IT'S SAFE TO SURRENDER IN SEX.

PS: I don't want sex. Sex is unavailable.
SEL: SINCE I KNOW I AM WANTED, I WANT SEX, AND IT IS ALWAYS AVAILABLE TO ME WHEN I WANT IT.

PS: I am not safe enough to ask for what I want sexually. I haven't a partner.
SEL: SINCE I KNOW I AM WANTED, I FEEL SAFE ENOUGH TO ASK FOR WHAT I WANT SEXUALLY, AND RECEIVE IT FROM THE NEW PARTNER I CREATED.

PS: I can't let go and relax and let my partner pleasure me.
SEL: SINCE I KNOW I AM WANTED, I CAN LET GO IN SEX AND LET MY PARTNER PLEASURE ME. PEOPLE WANT TO PLEASURE ME.

PS: I am a slow starter and a fast finisher.
SEL: SINCE I KNOW I AM WANTED, IT IS EASY FOR ME TO GET STARTED IN SEX, AND TO WAIT FOR MY PARTNER TO BE SATISFIED.

PS: I can't see my sexual desires as valid, or express them.
SEL: SINCE I KNOW I AM WANTED, I KNOW MY SEXUAL DESIRES ARE VALID AND I CAN EXPRESS THEM.

PS: I don't want sex when my partner wants sex.
SEL: SINCE I KNOW I AM WANTED, I CAN ALLOW MYSELF TO BE WANTED BY MY PARTNER SEXUALLY.

PS: I am not always present in sex. I have pain, and I don't orgasm.
SEL: SINCE I KNOW I AM WANTED, IT IS SAFE TO BE PRESENT IN SEX, AND IT IS PLEASURABLE TO ORGASM.

PS: I am closed and switched off. I can't get what I want.
SEL: SINCE I KNOW I AM WANTED AND I DESERVE WHAT I WANT IN SEX, I STAY OPEN AND TURNED-ON, IN ORDER TO GET WHAT I WANT.

PS: My husband died when I surrendered to being wanted by him.
SEL: SINCE I KNOW I AM WANTED, I AND MY PARTNER ARE SAFE WHEN I SURRENDER TO BEING WANTED SEXUALLY.

PL: I Can't Make It

PS: I don't want sex and I don't enjoy sex.
SEL: SINCE I KNOW I CAN MAKE IT, I WANT SEX AND I CAN ENJOY SEX.

PS: I can't let go and surrender in sex. If I let go, I will be trapped, or I won't survive.
SEL: SINCE I KNOW I CAN MAKE IT, THE MORE I LET GO IN SEX, THE SAFER AND MORE ALIVE I FEEL, AND THE MORE FREEDOM I HAVE.

PS: I am inadequate in sex.
SEL: SINCE I KNOW I CAN MAKE IT, I AM MORE THAN ADEQUATE SEXUALLY.

PS: I can't do sex right.
SEL: SINCE I KNOW I CAN MAKE IT, I CAN HAVE SEX BE COMPLETELY BLISSFUL AND PERFECT.

PL: I Don't Want to Be Here.

PS: If I surrender in sex, I will die.
SEL: SINCE I DO WANT TO BE HERE, THE MORE I SURRENDER IN SEX, THE MORE I WANT TO BE HERE AND THE MORE ALIVE I FEEL.

PS: I get emotionally involved with my partner when I have sex.
SEL: SINCE I KNOW I WANT TO BE HERE, IT'S SAFE TO GET EMOTIONALLY INVOLVED WITH MY PARTNER WHEN HAVING SEX.

PS: I don't let myself be sexually alive.
SEL: SINCE I KNOW I WANT TO BE HERE, IT'S SAFE TO BE SEXUALLY ALIVE.

PL: I Am Guilty.

PS: I hurt my partner in sex.
SEL: SINCE I KNOW I AM INNOCENT, I ONLY PLEASURE PEOPLE WITH MY SEXUAL ALIVENESS.

PS: There is not any sex, and if there is sex, it is not intimate enough.
SEL: SINCE I KNOW I AM INNOCENT, I HAVE ALL THE INTIMATE SEX I WANT.

PS: I deny myself sex if other parts of my life aren't working.
SEL: SINCE I KNOW I AM INNOCENT, I CAN HAVE AS MUCH LOVE, SEX AND MONEY AS I WANT.

PS: It's not safe to be intimate.
SEL: SINCE I KNOW I AM INNOCENT, INTIMACY IS SAFE FOR ME AND MY PARTNER.

PS: I am turned-on by both men and women.
SEL: SINCE I KNOW I AM INNOCENT, I AM INNOCENT FOR BEING TURNED-ON BY BOTH MEN AND WOMEN.

PS: I am not satisfied in sex.
SEL: SINCE I KNOW I AM INNOCENT, I DESERVE TO BE COMPLETELY SATISFIED SEXUALLY.

PS: I can't have the sexual partner I want.
SEL: SINCE I KNOW I AM INNOCENT, I CAN HAVE THE SEXUAL PARTNER I WANT.

PL: I Hurt People.

PS: Sex leads to intimacy, and then someone will be hurt.
SEL: SINCE I KNOW I PLEASURE PEOPLE, THE MORE INTIMATE I BECOME, THE MORE SEXUAL PLEASURE MY PARTNER AND I ENJOY.

PS: I don't let myself go enough to have pleasure, because I hurt people when I get what I want.
SEL: SINCE I KNOW MY ALIVENESS PLEASURES PEOPLE, THE MORE SEXUALLY ALIVE I AM, AND THE MORE I PLEASURE MYSELF, THE MORE I PLEASURE MY PARTNER.

PS: Bodies get in the way in sex.

SEL: SINCE I KNOW THAT I PLEASURE PEOPLE WITH MY ALIVENESS AND MY BODY, BODIES, BOTH MINE AND MY PARTNER'S, ENHANCE OUR PLEASURE IN SEX.

PL: I Am Useless.

PS: I have a guilty partner who doesn't enjoy sex.

SEL: SINCE I KNOW THAT I AM USEFUL AND INNOCENT, MY PARTNER FEELS INNOCENT ABOUT SEX, AND ENJOYS IT MORE AND MORE.

PS: The pleasure gets too great, and then I stop my sexual aliveness and get disappointed.

SEL: SINCE I KNOW I AM USEFUL, IT'S SAFE TO HAVE LOTS OF PLEASURE IN SEX. SEX IS ALWAYS A WONDERFUL SURPRISE.

PL: I Don't Belong.

PS: I climax too quickly and my interest fades.

SEL: SINCE I KNOW THAT I BELONG, MY SEXUAL ENERGY AND INTEREST LASTS AS LONG AS I WANT IT TO.

PL: I am Evil.

PS: I can't please myself.

SEL: SINCE I KNOW I AM PURE AND INNOCENT, I CAN PLEASE MYSELF.

PS: I can't let go, I can't relax, I can't receive what I want.

SEL: SINCE I KNOW I AM PURE AND INNOCENT, IT IS SAFE TO LET GO IN SEX. I CAN RELAX AND RECEIVE WHAT I WANT SEXUALLY.

PS: I go unconscious in sex.

SEL: SINCE I KNOW I AM PURE AND INNOCENT, IT'S SAFE TO BE 100% CONSCIOUS DURING SEX.

PL: I Am a Burden.

PS: I am not getting any sex.
SEL: SINCE I KNOW THAT I AM A GIFT, I RECEIVE ALL THE SEX I WANT.

PL: I Am Separate.

PS: I have a lack of intimacy in sex.
SEL: SINCE I KNOW THAT I AM CONNECTED, IT IS SAFE TO BE INTIMATE WITH MY SEXUAL PARTNER.

PS: I can't last long enough sexually with my partner.
SEL: SINCE I KNOW I AM CONNECTED WITH MY PARTNER, I KNOW THAT I CAN SATISFY MY PARTNER AND LAST AS LONG AS I WANT SEXUALLY.

PL: I Am a Failure.

PS: I don't go for it in sex because I will fail.
SEL: SINCE I KNOW I AM A SUCCESS, I CAN GO FOR IT SEXUALLY BECAUSE I AM A SEXUAL SUCCESS.

PS: I will kill someone in sex.
SEL: SINCE I KNOW I AM A SUCCESS, MY SEXUALITY IS A SUCCESS IN PLEASING, PLEASURING AND ENHANCING MY PARTNER'S ALIVENESS.

PL: I Am Bad.

PS: I judge myself for liking kinky sex.
SEL: SINCE I KNOW I AM GOOD AND PURE, EVERYTHING I LIKE SEXUALLY IS GOOD, PURE AND INNOCENT.

PS: Pleasure does not evolve.
SEL: SINCE I KNOW I AM GOOD AND PURE, SEX EVOLVES EASILY AND WITH PLEASURE.

PL: I Am Horrible.

PS: I hate men's penises. They are horrible.
SEL: SINCE I KNOW I AM WONDERFUL, I NOW FIND MEN'S PENISES WONDERFUL.

PS: I Am Not Perfect.

PS: I can't let go in sex.
SEL: SINCE I KNOW I AM PERFECT, IT'S SAFE TO LET GO IN SEX.

PS: I can't get what I want.
SEL: SINCE I KNOW I AM PERFECT, I CAN GET WHAT I WANT SEXUALLY.

PL: I Am Wrong.

PS: I can't please myself.
SEL: SINCE I KNOW I AM RIGHT, I KNOW THE RIGHT WAY TO PLEASE MYSELF, AND I CAN PLEASE MYSELF.

PL: I Am Invisible.

PS: I have to perform sexually to be remembered.
SEL: SINCE I KNOW THAT I AM VISIBLE AND NOTICED, I NO LONGER HAVE TO PERFORM SEXUALLY TO BE LOVED AND REMEMBERED.

PL: I Am Nothing.

PS: There is no sex.
SEL: SINCE I KNOW I AM EVERYTHING, I CAN HAVE AS MUCH SEX AS I LIKE WITH MY INTIMATE PARTNER.

PL: I Am Unwanted as a Woman.

PS: I have to hurry up sex, and I don't get what I want.
SEL: SINCE I AM WANTED AS A WOMAN, I CAN HAVE WHAT I WANT SEXUALLY, AND TAKE AS MUCH TIME AS I WANT.

PL: I Am Not Good Enough as a Man.

PS: I feel unwanted sexually, and not OK for being gay.
SEL: SINCE I AM GOOD ENOUGH AS A MAN, I AM WANTED SEXUALLY AS A MAN, AND I APPROVE OF MYSELF FOR BEING GAY.

After reading how other people's Personal Lies and biggest problems with sex connect, look at your own situation.

1. My Personal Lie, or most negative thought about myself, is ________.

2. The biggest problem I have with sex is ________.

3. My Sexual Eternal Law:

Since I know that I am ________, I can now ________ sexually.

My Father's Side of the Story

Rhonda, our beloved "baby daughter," did tell it like it was—with one important omission . . . .

Gloria and I had an ideal happy marriage. After a rocky start—I was just out of my teens and Gloria was a teenager—we overcame all obstacles and predictions, and made our union work.

We had two lovely daughters, Arlene and Ellen, and after almost ten years we decided to try and see if we could produce a son. Both Gloria and I kept reassuring each other, "We don't care about the sex of the baby in your womb; please God make 'it' healthy, with all of the proper equipment."

All of our children were born at home with natural childbirth procedures. As our third child emerged, I assisted with the pressure and the counting, and helped our M.D. bring the new baby out.

For just a fleeting moment—and that's all it was, Rhonda—I felt a sinking thud—which quickly changed to joy as I counted the ten fingers, ten toes, two eyes, etc. Both mother and I were thrilled. You were a beautiful, healthy baby! And we were overjoyed to have you!

I never thought of you as a boy, although I appreciated your going to baseball and football games with me. I was never a male chauvinist, and my three daughters made me a leading cheerleader for women's rights. In fact, I belong to the League of Women Voters.

Rhonda, you are your own self, and we thank God that you are interested in helping others seek happiness through the Loving Relationships Training. We love you, and wish you continued success.

CHAPTER 4

Infancy & Childhood

Infancy and Sex

THE IMPORTANT THING to remember when reading this chapter is that everything that happened to us in our infancy, every touch we received, every reaction we felt to our sexuality, we remember in our subconscious minds. We have stored these memories of our first touch, bonding with our mothers and fathers, feeding, toilet training, holding, and nurturing, to be triggered off as results when we create intimate experiences with our partners.

There are many factors in our infant lives which effect our sexuality. How the people at our birth react to whether we are a girl or a boy effects how we feel about our sexuality. There is a lot of confusion around sexuality. This sexual confusion often starts right at birth, when the baby comes out. If the baby feels disappointment, or anything other than complete joy around his or her sexuality, s/he could become sexually confused.

How the baby is touched right at birth is an important factor in how this being likes to be touched sexually as an adult. The baby at birth is vulnerable and naked, and has never before been touched by human hands. If the touching is rough, or if the baby is treated as an object when s/he is cleaned or touched, s/he may decide touching doesn't feel good, or it hurts.

The womb is a very sensuous environment, and the baby is nurtured by its warm water and soft walls. On his or her skin is a waxy substance called "vernix," which protects and insulates the baby. When s/he is born, the vernix is cleaned off. If this is done unconsciously or roughly, the baby's first response to touch can be quite negative. Also, at this time the baby is weighed on a cold scale, measured, and the cord is cut. All these events cause the baby to make decisions about life outside the womb.

If the baby's cord is cut too quickly or roughly, the baby may decide breathing is painful. The first breath was painful, so breathing is painful. These babies may unconsciously hold their breath whenever they are in a new or fearful situation. Often people hold their breath when having sex. The more we breathe, the more pleasure there is in sex. This pattern of holding one's breath starts right at birth with the cutting of the cord. Sex brings up birth issues and vulnerability. Sex is really enhanced when people let go of fear, and breathe.

The bonding period between mother, father and baby is also an important time. This is when the choice is made between feeling separate or feeling connected to other human beings.

When my children were born they were cuddled, loved, talked to, and made to feel welcome as soon as they came out, by both my husband and myself. Raynbow, my oldest child, had her grandparents, aunt, and some of our close friends there to celebrate her arrival. Jarrett, my second child, had his sister Raynbow, his parents, grandparents and other friends to welcome him to the world. My children love being around other children, family and friends. They feel very connected and safe with people.

Since I had a home birth for both my children, and I also was delivered at home, I had a strong belief that birth was about being connected and bonded to my parents, and I passed this belief on to my children. My children had Leboyer births. This is a gentle birthing practice geared toward complete comfort and gentleness for the baby. There is a lot of sensitivity about being quiet, having low lights, and keeping the environment as similar to the womb as possible. The baby is allowed to go at his or her own pace. S/he is not held upside down and spanked. S/he is gently put on the mother's belly to be held, and hear the mother's heartbeat like s/he did in the womb. S/he is allowed to start to breathe on his or her own before the umbilical cord is cut.

Once the cord is cut, he is put in warm water which is the same temperature as the womb. When he is put in the water, he usually smiles, remembering his fond memories of the womb. Both my husband and father held my children in the water, and this added to their sense of bonding and connection. Babies usually look up at whomever is holding them. Everything about this type of birth is about welcoming the child to the world in a gentle and loving way. These babies feel a lot of trust and safety in their relationships later on in life. They expect to be treated in a loving, supportive way.

Many babies are born in hospitals and separated from their mothers right away. The decision they make is that they have to be separate to survive.

When these people get into intimate relationships, they find it hard to be bonded and connected to their partners, especially after the intimacy of sex.

People can now have a hospital birth or a birth at a Birth Center, where the baby rooms in, and never leaves the mother. Even hospitals see the value in this early bonding period for the well-being of the baby.

There used to be a belief that babies didn't know anything until they were six months old. If babies smiled before six months, mothers were told they had gas and were not smiling. Now we all know better, and the medical profession is slowly but surely realizing that babies are aware and conscious at birth.

Dr. Leboyer played a very significant role in turning the medical profession around with his book, *Birth Without Violence*. After delivering 10,000 babies while believing babies didn't feel or know anything at birth, he had an enlightening experience. As a baby he was delivering was crowning, he realized that the baby was totally conscious and aware of everything happening to it. At this point he felt guilt for having delivered 10,000 babies while thinking they didn't know what was going on, and for treating them in an unenlightened way. Then he developed his gentle birthing practice described earlier.

In the old days, babies were only brought to their mothers at feeding time. They would be connected at feeding time, then they would be separated again and taken back to the nursery. Feeding time became the only time for love, affection and nourishment. Often these hospital babies were put on a four-hour schedule, so they only had food, love and affection every four hours.

The decision these babies made was that they had to wait for food, pleasure and affection, and after they received it, they had to be separate. In relationships, these people could feel connected during sex, and then abruptly become separate. They could act that out by jumping out of bed, or leaving after sex. They are not used to being intimate and connected after they are nurtured. Sex in this situation becomes like the food they received when they were brought to their mothers. It's only OK to be connected for as long as it takes to eat or to have sex.

How the baby is fed is very important to her early conditioning around sexuality. As already mentioned, feeding equals nurturing. Later in life, nurturing often becomes sexual nurturing. How you are nurtured as a baby affects your ability to receive nurturing as an adult. If you were breastfed by your mother, the decision was "I can get what I want". In breastfeeding, there is a very close bond between mother and child, which is very alive and connected. The baby is usually held closely, touched, and talked to in a loving way. Breasts are also sexual and sensuous. There is pleasure for both the mother and child in this process.

If a baby is bottlefed, he can still be loved and nurtured during this time. However, most often the decision bottlefed babies make is "I can't have what I want, because I really wanted my mother's breast to nurture me".

People who were only nursed for a short time, could feel later on that they get what they want for a short time, and then lose it. They could constantly be getting what they want in sex for a short time, and then losing their partners, or losing the drive to have what they want. Their thought is that they couldn't keep what they wanted. Often women stop breastfeeding because they are told they don't have enough milk to nourish their babies. When these babies are grown, they may get the nourishment or sex they want, but don't feel satisfied because it isn't the way they wanted it.

Men who were not nursed may have an obsession with big-breasted women. The men I have interviewed who were not breastfed often admit they are attracted to, and obsessed with, thoughts of being with big-breasted women. If they have sex with women with small breasts, they are disappointed, and feel they can't have what they want. The obsession with big breasts occurs because to an infant, the mother's breast looks really big!

The breastfed man is usually turned on to breasts, but he is also turned on to women's faces, legs, and other parts of the feminine body. The obsession with big breasts just doesn't seem to be there for men who were satisfied as babies by being breastfed. Also, whether an infant was fed on demand or on a schedule is important to the decisions made about nourishment, sex, affection, and even money. Babies that are fed on demand, or whenever they are hungry, usually have the thought, "I can have what I want when I want it." This can apply to sex, money, food, love, and affection.

My experience with nursing my two children was that in the beginning, sometimes they liked to be fed a little every thirty minutes to one hour. This was their way of connecting with me and being nurtured. Since in the womb they were connected all the time, they wanted to re-establish their connection with me, and assure themselves they could have what they wanted from me.

Scheduled feeding means that the baby is fed usually every four hours. If the baby is hungry in one hour, s/he has to wait for three more hours before being fed. The thought is, "I can't have what I want when I want it. I have to wait to get what I want." Often people who were fed on schedule feel addicted to not having what they want when they want it. They feel they always have to wait and be patient to receive gratification, whether it's sex, food, money, love or affection.

If two people in a relationship were fed differently as infants, this can affect their relationship. The person who was fed on demand may appear too demanding about wanting sex, love, or affection from their partner, who was schedule-fed, and feels you must wait to receive what you want.

This dynamic can create struggle and upset, because these two people are out of sync in their timing and their decisions about life. Until the schedule partner changes his thoughts to, "I can have what I want when I want it, and it's OK for my partner to have what s/he wants when s/he wants it", there could be constant struggle in the relationship. The demand partner will go for what s/he wants, and the schedule partner will resent him for wanting it, and expecting it, because s/he couldn't have it that way as a baby.

I was a demand baby, and I had a relationship with a man who was a schedule baby. We were always fighting and arguing about everything. We were both invested in being right about our own way of doing things. If I wanted to eat lunch at twelve o'clock, he would tell me I had to wait, or I could wait. When I would say, ". . . but I want it now", he would always say I was very demanding. I now see that he expected to have to wait, and that made him resent me for getting what I wanted so easily. These fights could happen about anything. If the demand partner wanted sex, the schedule partner might say you have to wait. A demand baby doesn't like to be told to wait, so s/he might become even more demanding, which ends up turning off both people.

Just like birth, sex is a very vulnerable time, with lots of holding, touching, kissing and connecting. Some people have a hard time really connecting and being present with their partners. If the mother is drugged during the birth, the baby will come out drugged, having received the drugs through the umbilical cord. As adults, these drugged babies often feel unconscious, drugged, or not present 100% when they are making love. They might feel like they need to have drugs to connect sexually with their partners. Since drugs are part of the birth script, they could feel they need to relive the drug experience over and over again through sex.

How the baby's genitals are treated by the nurse or parents is important for later decisions about his or her sexuality. If the parent or nurse cleans the genitals roughly, or ignores it, the baby may make the decision that their genitals are bad. Also, right at birth, the baby's genitals are covered up with a diaper. Right at birth, babies "get" that it's not OK to show their genitals. Actually, babies love to be diaperless. My babies were always pulling their diapers off to run around nude. Somewhere around two years, they become more shy and less innocent about showing their nude genitals.

Diaper changing is a very important time for a baby to make decisions about their sexuality. If the mother is embarrassed or shows any negative feelings when diapering the baby, the decision made by the baby could be, my genitals embarrassed my mother, they are not OK, they are bad, they are not something people like to see or touch. If the baby is stroked and touched lovingly when diapered, the decision would be that it is OK to have genitals, my genitals are pleasurable, and people like me to have pleasure.

Later on, toilet training is an important learning time. Since genitals are associated with elimination, as well as sexual and sensuous feelings, how toilet training is handled can effect the baby's decisions about his or her sexuality.

If toilet training is presented as a natural process that is innocent and easy, the child will not make any negative decisions about his genitals and toilet training. However, if a big deal is made in a negative way, with the parent conveying that this is dirty and bad, and you are bad when you aren't toilet trained, the child may also feel that their genitals are dirty and bad.

If toilet training is forced too early on the baby, they may be compulsively clean later in life, and feel that no matter what they do, their genitals are still dirty and bad.

Bathing is a pleasurable, sensual experience for the baby. How bathing is treated by the mother and father is also important in the formation of thoughts about bodies, and whether the baby decides her body is pleasurable and innocent, or not.

Often little boy babies have erections when bathed in soothing, warm water. The warm water is sexual and pleasurable, and reminds the boy of the womb which he loved. If the parents react negatively to the baby's pleasure, he may decide it is wrong to be fully alive and have sexual pleasure. He may decide that pleasure is not safe, and he might feel guilty for receiving pleasure as an adult.

Little girl babies also love to touch their genitals a lot. If the mother or father takes their baby's hand away and says "no", she may decide it's not OK to touch her genitals, or receive pleasure from them. Right at this point in infancy, the baby could shut down sexually, and not touch herself again to give herself pleasure until adult life.

I waited until college to experiment with masturbation. I must have touched myself often as an infant, and gotten disapproval from my father or mother, who always bathed me. I shut down, and didn't allow myself pleasure from myself until I was frustrated that I couldn't have orgasms and pleasure with my boyfriend. At this point, I decided to learn about myself again by exploring, and seeing what I wanted sexually. It took me quite a long time to let go of guilt about touching myself. As I became more innocent about touching myself, I was able to discover what gave me pleasure. The more innocent I felt, the more I let go and relaxed, and the more pleasure I received.

How much you were touched, tickled, and played with as an infant would also influence how you feel about being touched and being affectionate. Some people have so much fear and embarrassment about sexuality, that they are afraid to show affection or receive affection from their partners in public. When interviewing people about whether their parents were affectionate in front of the children, I found a direct correlation between this, and whether or not the same people felt comfortable showing affection in public. The adults who had never seen their parents acting affectionately toward each other when they were growing up, said they had a hard time being affectionate in public.

It's amazing that we have so much going on in the first two years of our lives that we don't consciously remember. These first two years are very important conditioning years for our sexuality and sensuality. The purpose of this chapter is to activate and stimulate your mind to start thinking about your infancy, and what decisions you made.

These decisions are about being a sexual being; experiencing pleasure; feeling pleasure is innocent; receiving what you want, how and when you want it; being touched and how that feels; feeling safe and connected to another human being. If you don't like the decisions you made in infancy, and thus the results you have in your life, you can choose out of them, and make other choices. At the end of this chapter, there are affirmations for changing negative decisions made in infancy.

Affirmations for the Infancy Period

1. I am a wonderful surprise as a man (woman).
2. It's safe to be a sexual man (woman).
3. Everyone is happy I am a girl (boy), and so am I.
4. Being a woman (man) is joyful.
5. It's safe to be vulnerable.
6. Every touch I receive is nurturing and loving.
7. Touching feels great, sexy and sensuous.
8. It's safe to be completely connected to my partner.

9. I can be 100% conscious and present in sex.
10. I am a welcome gift.
11. It feels good to touch my genitals.
12. It's safe and innocent to touch my genitals.
13. My genitals bring me pleasure.
14. The pleasure I receive from my genitals is innocent.
15. My elimination processes are easy, safe and normal.
16. My genitals are clean.
17. I can have what I want when I want it.
18. I can have what I want when I want it, and so can my partner.
19. My partner wants me to have what I want when I want it.
20. My breasts and vagina are beautiful and give me pleasure.
21. My penis is beautiful and gives me pleasure.
22. It's right to have sexual pleasure.
23. It's innocent to have sexual pleasure.
24. Being affectionate in public is normal and natural.

The Oedipal Period of Exploring Sex (Ages 4 to 6)

Sigmund Freud called the time from four to six, the Oedipal Period. This is an extremely sexual age for children. In my research and experience as a pre-school teacher, this is the age when children really explore and discover their sexuality, realizing the differences between boys and girls. This is also the period when a lot of incest occurs between children and their parents, and between siblings.

I was a pre-school teacher for six years, and I had the opportunity to observe children quite a bit. When I was first teaching, I worked in a college pre-school laboratory, which was set up with one-way mirrors in order to observe the children at play. We could watch them without their knowing we were there. The little girls would lift up their skirts and examine their genitals, and the little boys would unzip their pants so the girls could see their penises. They would also experiment with kissing each other, and touching each other's genitals. They would call it "playing house"; they were imitating their parents.

The four and five year olds also loved to play doctor, and the favorite examining area was their genitals. The children were always quite innocent in their play, but they would be embarrassed if they were caught. It was a lot of fun to watch the children play house, because they would act out their parents' relationships, or their perceptions of their parents. This also gave us, as teachers, great insights into their family life.

I remember being in Seattle for a one-month leadership program Sondra Ray and Fred Lehrman were leading. A woman from London had her four-year-old daughter with her. This little girl would constantly sit in the center of the group, lift up her dress, and masturbate in front of the whole group. She was very innocent about it, however, her mother was quite embarrassed. Children often act out the minds of their parents. The girl was acting out the sexual suppression her mother was feeling as a result of being away from her boyfriend for a month.

Often, this is the age when boys and girls stop taking baths together, and mothers stop bathing little boys because they have erections in the bath. This is an important time of conditioning about sex. If children are disapproved of or punished for their sexuality, they can become extremely guilty about it. Later in life, this could cause them to be really suppressed sexually. As pre-school teachers, when we came upon children exploring their sexuality, we just turned the other way, in order to allow them their innocence and privacy.

Sometimes at this age children will actually experiment with intercourse. There is usually a lot of masturbation unless parents stop it, and siblings of the opposite sex, and even the same sex, will explore each other.

Since kids are so sexual at this age, a little girl sitting in her father's lap could cause him to get an erection. He could feel guilty, take her off his lap with no explanation, and never allow her to sit there again. When there is no communication, she feels she is losing her father's love and affection. This is a turning point for many girls, who make the decision, "I can't have affection and love from my father, the man I love and want." If mothers will no longer bathe their sons, little boys can make the decision, "I can't have love and affection from my mother, the woman I really love."

Both girls and boys hook up their sexual feelings and aliveness with the loss of their parents' affection. They usually suppress both their feelings and their sexuality until they grow up. The thoughts of not being able to have the one you want sexually will emerge later in life, when you are with a partner you really love. The children will shut down their sexuality and their innocence because the reactions they received made them believe their sexuality was wrong and bad.

A lot of acted-out incest occurs at this age between fathers and daughters. Little girls of four often have more sexual energy than their mothers. They unknowingly turn on their fathers. If the father is alcoholic or emotionally weak, he could act out the incest. The same thing is true for mothers and sons.

A client of mine started remembering some sexual incidents she had had with her father at the age of four. The memories started to surface in dreams, hypnosis, and rebirthing. She didn't remember anything consciously, but she had extreme sexual guilt. She had become a nun at sixteen in order to get away from her alcoholic father, and suppress her sexual guilt. The actual memory finally came to her when she had a thigh massage. Her father had fondled her when she was on his lap. He had had an erection, and felt guilty and embarrassed. She had taken on his guilt, and shut down her sexuality. She became a nun, and later, after she left the convent, she became a homosexual. She no longer trusted men.

Often parents will give their children enemas at this age, which is also very sexual. I know a man whose mother gave him enemas when he was four and five. He felt sexually abused and manipulated by her. As an adult, he had an extreme fear of being controlled and manipulated sexually by women.

From four to six, boys and girls really show an interest in the opposite sex. They kiss, touch, and have boyfriends and girlfriends. After about six, there seems to be an aversion to the opposite sex. Boys hate girls and vice versa. Boys play with boys, and girls play with girls. Between six and eleven, there seems to be low sexual energy in children. When they reach puberty, their sexual energy is back on the rise, and there is a re-kindled interest in the opposite sex.

The purpose of this chapter is to stimulate any memories you have about your sexuality at this age. If you shut down sexually during this period because of something that happened to you, or because of a reaction from your parents to something you did, you can change your mind now, and assume again your childhood innocence and exploration of your sexuality.

Childhood Incidents of Sexuality—the Oedipal Period

DANIEL

When I was .... four or five, I touched my mother's breast and she got angry, and would not allow it. Between the ages of two and four, my mother reprimanded me for touching my penis, and told me that if I didn't stop, she would call a doctor she knew to cut it off.

The decision I made about my sexuality from these incidents was .... I was bad, guilty and would be punished if I pleasured myself.

VIVIENNE

When I was ... four, I started to masturbate. My mother told me that I would go blind if I continued to masturbate.

The decision I made about my sexuality from this incidents was .... I started to wear glasses as a child because I continued to masturbate behind my parents' back.

MATHEW

When I was .... four, I played around with my four girl cousins. I knew I better not get caught. I got caught, and my parents sent me to an all-boy's school when I was five.

The decision I made about my sexuality from these incident was .... I get punished for having pleasure. I still have a hard time having pleasure with a woman.

JOHN

When I was .... four, I was riding a tricycle with a little girl, and I had an erection.

The decision I made about my sexuality from this incident was .... that girls were different and exciting.

BEN

When I was .... four, I had a bathtub scene with a little girl my age. I noticed thinking that the little girl must have had her penis cut off.

The decision I made about my sexuality from this incident was .... Either girls were different, or I had better not do anything bad or I might get my penis cut off.

SHARDA

When I was . . . . four, I noticed a boy had a penis. I thought he was different than me, and he had something extra.

The decision I made about my sexuality from this incident was . . . . Girls and boys were different, and boys have more than girls.

MISA

When I was . . . . four or five, a man played with me inside my pants. It felt exhilarating.

The decision I made about sexuality from this incident was . . . . Good girls don't do this or enjoy this: if you enjoy it you get guilty.

JOHN PAUL

When I was . . . . five, I was playing house with a little girl outside of my house. My father saw me and called me a pervert, and said my behavior was inappropriate.

The decision I made about my sexuality from this incident was . . . . Being interested in girls would lead to disapproval. As I grew up, I had inappropriate sexual experiences that caused embarrassment.

JANEY

When I was . . . . three, something happened with my father; he withdrew sexually from me. I found out about death at age four, and shut down my sexuality at age three.

The decision I made about my sexuality from this incident was . . . . That I can not have the attention and affection from the man I want.

The Puberty Period (Ages 11 to 14)

Usually in the sixth grade, boys and girls start to have a keen interest in the opposite sex, just as they did in the Oedipal Period. Often people do not remember exploring sex from four to six, and their first conscious memories of their sexuality are of puberty.

My daughter, who is now thirteen, had boyfriends in nursery school and kindergarten, hated boys from first grade through fifth grade, and then all of a sudden in sixth grade was interested in boys again. She went steady, went to mixed parties, and played kissing games.

Puberty is a very sensitive time of discovery of our sexuality and sensuality. Both boys and girls have feelings in their bodies they have never felt before. Pre-teen moods shift up and down like a roller coaster. They feel totally at the affect of their hormonal changes.

Puberty was a crossroads for me. I had fooled myself into believing I was a boy to please my father; I had been a total tomboy. I had not let my body develop in a feminine way. All my friends were developing breasts, and I was flat as a board. I finally convinced my mother I should buy a bra, even though I had nothing to put in it. She consented, and suggested I should get one with pads, so it looked like I had some breasts. I was really embarrassed when the rumor went around my class that I wore falsies. I took off the bra, and decided to go back to being a tomboy.

When I was twelve and a half, after a new Year's Eve slumber party with my girlfriends where we stayed up all night, I got my period for the first time. I was really afraid I had done something horrible or bad, and this was my punishment. My mother had never explained menstruation to me because my sisters did not menstruate until they were fourteen, and she didn't expect me to be so early.

Since she had not warned me in advance, I walked around in my dirty underwear feeling guilty and bad. Finally, I confessed to my mother something terribly wrong had happened to me. She laughed and slapped my face. She said slapping my face was a Jewish custom for welcoming me into womanhood. I felt I was being punished for being a woman by having this horrible thing called menstruation, and it felt like a slap in the face or a humiliation to be a woman. I still didn't want to be a woman, and my breasts really didn't grow until I was in college.

Often, when a girl starts to develop, her father gets embarrassed, gets an erection when she walks across the room, and withdraws his love and affection out of embarrassment. Boys start to look more like men, reminding their mothers of their husbands in younger days. Mothers can also feel excited around their sons, get embarrassed, and withdraw their love and affection.

Incest patterns, both suppressed and acted out, get activated during puberty. Many acted-out incest situations occur between fathers and daughters, or mothers and sons, at this time. If the incest is acted out, there is both pleasure and guilt. Often, it is really scary for an eleven-to-fourteen year old to have their sexual feelings aroused, and they feel really guilty if the sex is acted on and they have pleasure. Later in life, they associate sexual pleasure with guilt. They usually make the decision that they are bad for having pleasurable sexual feelings.

Because of all the sexual feelings eleven-to-fourteen year olds have, they draw sexual attention to themselves from their parents, step-parents and other adults. Often, rapes occur at this age as well.

All children and their parents have suppressed sexual feelings for each other. Children want the love and affection of their parent of the opposite sex. If they don't get the love and affection of that parent, they decide "I can't have the man or woman I want for love, affection, or sex." If they do get the sexual attention they want from the parent, they usually pick up the parent's guilt. Then they feel bad, dirty, and guilty for getting the attention they wanted.

Look back to your puberty, and try to remember how you felt about the opposite sex. Try to recall how you felt about the changes going on in your body. What kind of attention or lack of attention did you receive from your parents about your changing body?

Incidents of Sexuality—The Puberty Period

PETRA

When I was . . . . twelve, I got my period. I thought that I was bleeding to death. No one had told me about menstruation. All my girlfriends teased me because I looked different, because I developed early.

ZAK

When I was . . . . eleven or twelve, I was climbing a rope in gym with the boys. I had an orgasm, and sperm came out all over my pants. All the boys laughed. When I was eight or nine, I used to fool around with the farm boys. I knew something was missing—the girls. I started to show my penis to girls. I had sex very early—when I was thirteen.

BEN

When I was . . . . fourteen, I had my circumcision. I feel like I left the planet at this time. A man did this, and I still have a hard time trusting men.

SHARDA

When I was . . . . twelve, I stopped playing house and doctor with little boys.

MISA

When I was . . . . twelve, I grew breasts. Three boys followed me home from school one day and touched my breasts—I got excited and ashamed. I kept my sexuality hidden from my dad so he would still love me. At this time, I also got afraid of boys, and had a push/pull around sex. I was interested and afraid at the same time.

RACHEL

When I was . . . . six or seven, I started an incestuous relationship with my uncle that lasted until I was fourteen. My uncle acted towards me the way I wanted my father to act towards me. I always had the fear of being caught.

CHRIS

When I was . . . . twelve, I was very Catholic, and went to confessions. I felt extremely guilty for masturbating around the ages of thirteen and fourteen. Since this age, I have never been able to let anyone see me pee.

What Teenagers Want to Learn about Sex from Their Parents

Recently, I interviewed my teenage daughter and some of her friends about what they would like to learn and be told about sex from their parents.

Teenagers are very wise, and we can learn a lot from them. They told me that sex education starts out when children are young, under the age of five.

This is when trust is established between parents and children concerning sexuality. If children ask questions, what they want from their parents is the truth. If the parents are too embarrassed to talk about sex to their children, they should admit their embarrassment, and then tell the truth as best they can. If parents don't tell the truth about where babies come from, how babies are made, and the biological differences between girls and boys, their children will know they are not being told the truth. Then they will look elsewhere to find out about sex, and they may receive misinformation.

One teenager I talked to said her parents avoided the topic of sex with her. She experimented with sex at twelve years old, because she was curious and wondered what it would feel like. As she was growing up, she never thought her parents had sex. However, she would go into the bathroom looking for toilet paper, and find sponges and other sexual items. She had a curiosity about what her parents were doing.

She found out about sex from friends, movies, books and teachers. She had a sister seventeen years older than she, who she asked questions about sex. Her sister told her how sex should and shouldn't be, about sexual diseases, and about taking responsibility for protecting herself against both disease and pregnancy. Her parents basically told her that it was up to her to make her own decisions about sex, based on knowing the facts and the consequences.

She also said she was disappointed that she had experimented with sex so young. What she did learn from being sexual was that she could say "no" to sex if she didn't want it. She has decided she wants sex in long-term relationships, rather than in short-term relationships or casual dating. She now feels that she would like to develop a friendship before having sex. She feels that boys drop you faster after you have sex, and she has a hard time maintaining a relationship after she has had sex.

Another girl said she would only talk about sex to her children if they asked her questions. She felt that it was the kids' choice of where, when and from whom they would learn about sex. She said she was too embarrassed to talk to adults about it. She feels more comfortable talking to her friends. She found out about it from her babysitter and books at age five. In sixth grade, she said she had a good sex education course in school where they had discussion groups. This class was beneficial in allowing her to make choices about sex based on the facts.

The girls felt that boys do pressure girls to have sex, but they have the right to say "no" if they don't want to do it. They also felt that boys were only interested in their own pleasure. They said they felt guilty, bad and dirty about having sex. One girl felt like she had sinned by having sex.

What these teenagers would tell their own children about sex is:

1. About sexual disease.
2. How to protect themselves from disease and pregnancy.
3. How to make a decision whether or not to be sexual, based on facts and the truth.
4. How to deal with peer pressure: how to say "no" when you don't want sex.
5. That having sex doesn't necessarily lead to popularity.
6. That having sex is not something to take lightly.
7. What they might expect in the sexual experience.

What these teenage girls felt about sex after their experimentation, was that sex was disappointing, painful, and heartbreaking. How they would like sex to be is passionate and wonderful, like it is in romance novels.

CHAPTER 5

Sexual Patterns & How They Affect Us

What Our Parents Told Us About Sex and Intimacy

OUR PARENTS HAD a more profound influence on us than anyone else. What they communicated to us verbally, by their actions, or what they didn't tell us about sex, affects our sexuality.

In the LRT, we spend a lot of time discussing and releasing ten patterns that affect us. A pattern is a form of repetitive, unconscious behavior. For example, if every time you reach nine months in your intimate relationships, you leave, this is described as a leaving pattern. A pattern is something you do over and over again unconsciously. We also unconsciously conform or rebel against our parents' minds.

Our minds thrive on familiarity. Since we probably lived between sixteen and twenty years with our parents, and what they did was familiar to us, then depending on how we felt about our parents, we either conform to, or actively rebel against, their actions, words, and minds. Whether we rebel or conform to our parents' minds, we are still at the affect of them.

Before I discuss how these patterns affect our sexuality, I want to let you know how to release them. The first step in releasing a pattern is to notice it operating in your life. The second step is to admit your addiction to it. The addiction is similar to being addicted to alcohol, drugs or food; in order to release it, you first have to say "Yes, I am an addict. Yes, I am addicted to copying my parents in the area of sexuality". The third step occurs when you are really sick of the pattern, usually after you have indulged in it. Then you can actively say "no" to it, and choose out.

The first three patterns we discuss in the LRT weekend describe how we use our parents as models in our intimate relationships. The first pattern is choosing an intimate partner who has a personality like one of our parents. The tendency is to choose a partner who is like the parent with whom you had the most trouble. For example, when I was growing up I had the most difficulty with my mother. I felt that she was a perfectionist, critical, and had a short fuse. She was also an Aries, very creative, a professional dancer, had a great laugh, and when she laughed, it was very infectious. My mother and I fought a lot, especially during my puberty.

I had a relationship with a man for three years who was exactly like my mother. He was critical, somewhat of a perfectionist, a professional dancer, an Aries, had a short fuse, and an infectious laugh. Needless to say, we had a lot of fights, just like my mother and I had had. We also had a lot of sex. We probably had sex every day for three years. The anger and upsets gave us a lot of energy to make-up and have sex. The sex seemed to be a release for the anger and tension that we had. We broke up after three years and never had sex again, and thank God we never fought again.

The reason we re-create partners like our parents is so that we can resolve our issues with our parents. When I was involved in this relationship, I realized how much unresolved anger and upset I had with my mother. I did the Forgiveness Diet on myself and my mother, and I wrote her completion letters. I was lucky because she also did LRTs; I was able to communicate verbally what I needed to in order to heal the relationship.

We use our partners to heal anything unresolved we have with our parents. As long as we realize that, and do what it takes to heal our relationship with our parents, we are able to have a better and better relationship with our intimate partner.

Pattern number two is creating a partner who treats us like our parent or parents treated us. An example for me happened after I had a tremendous healing with my mother. I no longer created a partner like her. I shifted to my father. I always felt I had a great relationship with my dad. However, in one relationship I had for about three months, I found out what I had unresolved with my father. When I was thirteen years old, my father commuted to Chicago for business for one year. If I was lucky, I saw him one weekend a month.

In this new relationship, I created my partner looking and acting like my father: good looking, charismatic, a good salesman, and having his business and money handled. The only problem was, like my father, he traveled a lot for business. He had never been to Chicago on business until he dated me.

He went there for business, and I was able to look at how much I hated not having my father there for me. The unresolved part of my relationship with my father was wanting him and not having him available for me. This relationship was very short-lived, because my partner traveled a lot in the three months we dated. We really didn't get to bond completely, and then he left for Africa for four months. He wrote me several times, and I considered myself still in the relationship.

Jeff and I got close as friends during this four-month period. About a week after he got back from Africa, my partner and I broke up. I was able to have a deeper healing with my father after this relationship. I also started to let go of my father more and more, so I could really let in a man who was completely there and available for me. Letting go enabled me to let in someone who was mine, and did not belong to my mother, his mother, or anyone else.

In this pattern, we might also act out the parent role, and treat our partner like our parents treated us. If your mother left, you might leave your partner in order to heal your relationship with your mother. You might also fear that your partner will leave you, so you leave first.

The third pattern is to copy our parents' relationship with each other. In other words, we relate to our partner just like our parents related to each other. So if our parents were affectionate only behind closed doors, this is how we would be with our partner. If our parents slept in separate beds or didn't have sex at all, we might copy them, and stop having sex with our partners.

Sometimes, what we think was the truth about our parents' sex life is only what we believed to be true. Our parents' sex life probably was, and is, better than we thought. For example, I thought my parents never had sex. They never talked about it; sex was really behind closed doors, and they had two twin beds next to each other. I assumed they didn't have sex. One day when I was a teenager, I came home late from a date, and caught my parents all curled up together in one bed, and I knew they had sex. I couldn't believed they actually "did it." Now at seventy-eight, my parents finally have a kingsize bed.

In my marriage, we rarely had sex. I really didn't want to. I didn't know how to have sex, or why anyone would want to. I can see now that I was copying what I thought had been my parents' sex life.

In summary, how we act out the first three patterns is through one of the following three laws which govern relationships. First, the law of attraction—we attract that which we are used to. For example, if a girl had a sexually abusive father, she attracts a sexually abusive partner. Second, the law of projection—you think your partner is acting like your parent, whether or not they really are. For example, your partner wants to be loving and sexual with you, and you see it as sexually abusive. Third, the law of manifestation—you drive your partner to be sexually abusive. Your partner is very loving and affectionate, but you keep pushing him away. He gets frustrated, and eventually starts to be rough and sexually abusive.

Another way you could act out this pattern sexually, is by attracting someone who treats you like your parents treated you physically. If your parents didn't give you any physical affection or touching, you could create a partner who doesn't touch you or give you affection. You could also create your partner giving you a lot of physical attention, but you interpret his or her behavior as unaffectionate. Or, s/he could be very physical and affectionate in the beginning, but because you expect him not to be affectionate, s/he stops being affectionate in order to live up to your expectations.

In order to get in touch with your thoughts about sex and intimacy, and how they relate to your parents' thoughts, do the following written processes.

My thoughts about sex are . . . .

My mother's thoughts about sex are . . . .

My father's thoughts about sex are . . . .

My thoughts about intimacy are . . . .

My mother's thoughts about intimacy are . . . .

My father's thoughts about intimacy are . . . .

Each chapter that precedes this one has its own affirmations. For this chapter, create your own affirmations by changing any negative thought you have about sex and intimacy. For example, if you think sex is a duty, the affirmation would be, "Sex is a pleasure for me and my partner."

Two main affirmations I want to give you for this chapter are:

1. It's safe to surpass my parents' sex life.
2. It's safe to surpass my thoughts about my parents' sex life.

A way to took at how you may be copying your parent's intimate relationship is to do the following written processes.

1. List ways your parents related to each other. Include intimately, sexually and physically.
2. List ways you have related to your present and most recent partners intimately, physically, and sexually.

Note the similarities, and notice if your relationships are the opposite of your parents' relationship, and you are rebelling from your parents' intimate relationship style. If you are happy with the way you relate, and it works for you, that's great. If not, then it's time to stop being at affect of your parents.

If you notice a lot coming up about your parents after reading this chapter, you could:

1. Write a completion letter to your parents. First, write a letter of upset or blame to them that you don't send. This will get the feelings out, and release the charge. Then, write a letter talking about your feelings and taking more responsibility. Use sentences like:

   I felt ________ when I saw you doing ________.

   I interpreted what you did as ________.

   How this affects my life now is ________.

When you would not mind receiving the letter you wrote, send it to your parent.

2. Do the Forgiveness Diet:

   I forgive myself 70 x 70.

   I forgive my mother 70 x 70.

   I forgive my father 70 x 70.

   I forgive my parents 70 x 70.

If you have a hard time completing with your parents on your own, get support. Call a rebirther, or take the Loving Relationships Training. In the LRT, a lot of time is spent clearing issues about our parents. Remember, you want to be your own person living in the moment, not a reflection of your parents, living in the past.

Sexual Secrets

Recently I was taking a workshop for women facilitated by fellow rebirther Jacquie McDonald. There I discovered that sexuality had always been kept secret in my family.

I can trace the beginning of the secrets back to my mother's conception, but I'm sure it goes back even further. My grandmother fell in love, and married an Italian. He spoke Hebrew and Yiddish fluently, and my grandmother assumed he was Jewish. Shortly after they were married, my mother was conceived. One day, my grandmother was going through her husband's trunk and found a crucifix. My grandmother was extremely religious; she was an Orthodox Jew. She was mortified that she had married a Catholic man. She had the marriage annulled, and denied the love and attraction she had for her husband.

My mother was born, and my grandmother remarried a Jewish man when my mother was under one year old. My mother always thought this man was her real father. When my mother was in her forties, she applied for a passport, and needed her birth certificate. She was shocked to find on the birth certificate that she was one year older than she had always thought, and that she had a different last name.

My mother repeated this pattern of secrecy in her own life unknowingly. She and my father met when they were very young—under eighteen. They fell in love and eloped, and kept the marriage secret from their families. They feared disapproval from their parents. They kept the marriage secret for one year—the time span between my mother's birth, and my grandmother's marriage to the man my mother always thought was her real father.

As my parents kept their sex life a secret from their parents in the beginning, so they also kept their sex life a secret from their children. It was as if I was supposed to believe my mother was a virgin. I felt when I was growing up that my parents never had sex. When I heard other kids talking about sex, I believed this was something that did not exist in my family. The truth was that my parents really loved each other, and were affectionate. I remember being shocked when I came home from a date in high school, and caught my parents in bed. I discovered my parents were sexual beings.

My parents were also very private about their bodies. I feel that all their children learned that our bodies were not to show to other people. We learned to be very private about our bodies. I know that I was embarrassed to be nude in front of both men and women. It took me quite a while to feel comfortable about my nude body.

This secrecy about sexuality affected me because my sexuality was kept a secret from me. My mother never talked to me about being a woman, or about the birds and the bees. I was very surprised when I got my period. I didn't know what it was, and I kept it a secret from my mother for a whole day. I finally told her, after I got scared that I might bleed to death. I thought I was being punished for something.

When I first had sex with my boyfriend in college, I kept it secret from my parents and almost everyone else. I had a Catholic roommate who discovered I was having sex, and believed that I was sinning. She called my father to let him know so that I would be punished. Then it was no longer a secret from my father that I was a woman, and a sexual being.

Since sex had always been hidden in both my life and my parents' marriage, I had a hard time enjoying sex when I was married. I was afraid of sex, and didn't want it. I also created my husband having secret affairs that he would tell me about a year afterwards.

Another thing I discovered in the workshop was that I kept my orgasms a secret, and I lied about having ones I didn't have. I started to have multiple orgasms when I was willing to tell the total truth about sex. It is important to know that you are good enough, and wanted enough, to deserve sexual pleasure on your own timetable. I used to be embarrassed that I would take a long time to achieve orgasm. I felt I would disappoint my partner if he had to wait a long time for me. Because I felt I was a disappointment as a woman, I set it up to feel like I would disappoint my partner if I really let myself wait to have pleasure for myself. This decision made me feel as though I had to fake orgasms, so I would please my partner instead of myself.

Now I tell the truth, and I don't keep it a secret if I am turned on and enjoying what my partner is doing to me. I even let him know what is feeling good. I usually let him know by sounds "ummmm, ahhhh, ooooh". I also let him know all my secret turn-on places that I discovered through masturbation. Jeffrey has one spot that he discovered that is still his secret spot to turn me on, to pleasure and please me.

What Sexual Secrets are there in your life? List all the sexual secrets kept from you. List all the sexual secrets you have kept from others.

Affirmations

1. It's safe to let go of all my sexual secrets.
2. It's safe to be truthful about my sexuality.
3. It's safe and easy to tell the truth about my pleasure.
4. The more I tell the truth in sex, the more orgasms and pleasure I have.
5. It's safe to reveal my sexuality.
6. The more I let my sexual energy out, the more energy I receive.

How Parental Disapproval Affects Our Sexuality

The Parental Disapproval Syndrome (PDS) is one of the most destructive patterns. It is the pattern which most diminishes our self-esteem. The lower our self-esteem, the less likely we are to be able to have a fulfilling, sexually intimate relationship.

PDS is handed down from one generation to another. Our parents were disapproved of by their parents, who had been disapproved of by their parents. Our parents didn't have a big enough vocabulary to stop their parents from disapproving of them. The outcome is that children give up their divinity to please their parents. Children are almost never allowed to have higher self-esteem than their parents.

Children are very alive and full of energy. If the parents were not allowed to express their aliveness in *their* parents' presence, they will do anything they can to stifle their own children's aliveness. They will say things like, "Don't make so much noise." and "Don't jump around." What they are really saying is, "Don't be so alive." Since as children we got disapproved of for being noisy, active and alive, we learn to stifle our aliveness in order to receive our parents' love.

Sexual energy is also aliveness. If as children we suppressed our aliveness, as adults we may also hold back our sexual aliveness. We do this out of habit—it is unconscious. We no longer remember what it is like to be children, and feel really alive.

We have to reclaim the divinity we lost as children. We have to again be the innocent, alive children of God we once were.

The reason we give in to PDS, is that this is the way we got attention from our parents. Maybe your father told you, "Don't put your tricycle in the driveway," and you listened. But then your father came home, read his newspaper, and didn't give you any attention. But when you put your trike in the driveway where he pulled his car in, he had to notice you. You may have thought that negative attention was better than no attention at all. For children, attention is extremely important, so if they don't get positive attention, they will settle for negative.

We tend to equate PDS, or disapproval, with love. As we grow up we become addicted to disapproval, because to us this means attention and love. We will attract a partner who disapproves of us. If we are really addicted to disapproval, and our partner doesn't disapprove of us, we will keep doing things they don't like in order to get our daily fix of disapproval. I remember getting frustrated once when my partner wouldn't disapprove of me. I kiddingly asked him for a spanking. I had not had enough of a dose of disapproval to satisfy my addiction. This is when I realized I didn't need it anymore.

If we have this pattern, and we don't create a partner to disapprove of us, we might create a boss to disapprove of us, or we might just disapprove of ourselves. Sexually, you might disapprove of yourself for not having orgasms, for not letting go, or for premature ejaculation. The more you disapprove of yourself, the worse it gets; the harder it gets to have an orgasm, let go, or sustain an erection.

Another way PDS might affect us sexually is that we might attract a partner who is disapproving of our ability as a lover. S/he might tell you that you are doing it wrong. Or, because you were disapproved of as a child, you might be a disapproving person yourself, and constantly disapprove of your mate.

Disapproval is not sexy. PDS does not turn on your partner. PDS distracts you from being sexual, and having bliss in your sex life.

You might even be in bed with your partner, and imagine that your parents are disapproving of you for having sex. Instead, imagine your parents in cheerleading outfits, cheering you on to bliss and orgasm.

Affirmations

1. I have now had enough disapproval in my life to know that I am loved.
2. I approve of and love myself unconditionally.
3. Everyone approves of my sexual aliveness.
4. I am a divine child of God.
5. My parents cheer me on to sexual bliss.
6. I approve of myself in my partner's presence.
7. I approve of my partner 100%.
8. I approve of myself for having sexual pleasure and orgasm.
9. I approve of my sex life just the way it is.
10. I approve of my sexual aliveness and energy.

Rebellion and Sexuality

The getting-even pattern is usually the reaction to, or outcome of, the PDS Pattern. Like me, most people who are rebels by nature have a revenge pattern going on.

Since we were disapproved of by our parents, and gave up our divinity, we take revenge on our partners or children. We take out our anger at our parents, on our partners, or children.

In this pattern, we are constantly striving to get even with our parents in our relationships. The truth is that you can never get even. You can only play the game of one-upsmanship. What happens is one person gets even, and then the other person gets even, and it keeps going on and on. What usually ends up happening is that we end up odd. We end up alone. Our partner gets tired of playing this game, and we get tired of getting new partners to act out our revenge with. Sometimes, we finally give up the revenge, because we realize that we no longer have anything to get even about.

I came out of the womb rebellious. Because my parents wanted a boy, and I was a girl, I turned in the womb and came out face up, the opposite of what my parents wanted. I basically came out saying "Fuck you, I am a girl, not a boy." I spent thirty-two years rebelling, and choosing the opposite of what I wanted, and what my parents wanted for me. They disapproved of me, and were disappointed momentarily that I was a girl, and I spent thirty-two years trying to get even with them.

I failed in my marriage in order to get even and prove they did a bad job. I failed in my job or career in order to prove they did a bad job. I ended up hurting myself more than I hurt my parents.

I failed in sex in order to get even with them. As you can see, we end up being the ones who get hurt. We end up getting even with ourselves, for believing we need to get even with our parents.

Because of this revenge pattern, I tried many ways to get even with my partners. I had affairs to get even. I talked behind a partner's back, to make him look bad, to get even. I left, to get even. I didn't have sex, or I withheld sex and affection, to get even. Withholding sex and affection can go back and forth between you and your partner, and create a pattern of resentment that blocks all the good feelings of sex.

To get in touch with your revenge pattern, do the following written process. List all the ways you have gotten even with your present and previous partners.

Forgive yourself for getting even with your partner, as revenge on your parents. I noticed that I wanted to get even with all men, because my dad didn't want me as a girl. I blamed all men, and took out my anger on people who didn't deserve it. Notice who you are angry at, and who you have been taking it out on.

It's safe to let go of revenge in order to have sex and intimacy be the way you want it to be. You will win in relationships when you give up the desire to get even. Getting rid of revenge gets you back in the present moment, which is the best time for sex.

Affirmations

1. The more my partner wins, the more I win. The more I win, the more my partner wins.

2. I am a winner in the area of sex and intimacy.
3. My partner is not my parent.
4. I forgive myself for thinking I had to get even with my parent(s).
5. My parents want me to win in relationships, and I want to win.
6. I want to win for me.
7. I am now even and happy.

Suppressed Family Sexuality

Have you ever been rejected in a relationship without knowing why?

Have you ever been attracted to, or involved with someone, who is already in a relationship, or married?

Have you ever been in a relationship, and had either you or your partner pull in a third person?

Have you ever been in a relationship where your partner seemed unavailable because they lived a long distance away?

Have you ever been in a relationship where your partner seemed unavailable because their work or hobby seemed more important to them than the relationship?

Have you ever had the sexual aspect of your relationship disintegrate or go flat when you felt connected and loving in other ways?

Have you felt uninterested in sex after you moved in with your partner?

Have you ever felt not sexually attracted to your partner after having a child, after it started to feel like family?

If you answered "yes" to one or more of the above questions, welcome to the very popular Club of Suppressed Family Sexuality-Incest. This club has about 90% or more of all the people I have ever met either participating in, or having participated in, one of the above situations, if not all of them.

The first time I ever heard of Suppressed Family Incest was in 1981, when I took the Loving Relationships Training. When Sondra Ray and Fredric Lehrman were discussing this issue, I went completely unconscious. What I mean by unconscious is that I was off daydreaming, thinking of other things;

physically in the room, but emotionally and intellectually somewhere else. I didn't hear a thing they said about incest, and I had no notes on the subject. I felt that it did not apply to me, that my father was not sexual with me, and I was certainly not attracted to him sexually. That was my definition of incest. I took the LRT several more times before I was able to be conscious and aware of what they were talking about. Of course, now that I am an LRT Trainer, I not only understand the incest pattern and teach it, I own it as one of the major patterns of my life that kept me from having the relationship I wanted.

Suppressed Family Incest means we wanted the love, affection and attention of our parents and siblings. We really wanted the love and affection of our family members of the opposite sex. Homosexuals wanted the love and affection of the parent of the same sex. The usual pattern is that our parents bathe us, cuddle us, tickle us, have us sit on their laps. Then suddenly, when we are somewhere between four and ten, they stop doing these things, and don't explain why. When they did these things to us, it felt really good. If an adult is tickled and touched like parents do to infants, the adult will get sexually aroused.

A boy's mother may have bathed him, tickled him, splashed him, washed him, etc.. One day he has an erection, his mother notices the erection, the boy notices his mother noticing, and the mother notices the boy noticing her noticing. She is embarrassed and leaves the bathroom, never to return again at bath time. She just tells her son he is old enough to bathe himself, with no other explanation. As long as the bath scene was innocent, it was OK for mom to participate, but as soon as the boy obviously received some sexual pleasure, it became not OK for her to be there. At this point, the mother withdraws her physical attention and affection from her son. This could happen when the boy is between the ages of three and six. This is described in an earlier chapter as the Oedipal Period, when children are first exploring and discovering their sexuality.

The bath scenario could also be a brother and sister bathing together. One day, the little boy has an erection and is ostracized from the bath and bathroom, never again allowed to take a bath with his sister. And probably he is given no explanation other than "you are too old to bathe together". My son and daughter use to bathe together. Raynbow is two years and nine months older than Jarrett. There was a point at which Raynbow refused to bathe with Jarrett, and wanted her privacy. She ostracized him from the bath. Either he had had an erection, or she started to feel embarrassed about being nude with her brother. This happened at the same time that they started fighting and arguing more.

Usually, little girls sit on their daddys' laps. These are very special moments, when little girls get their daddys' full love, attention, and affection. Most little girls are the "apple of their daddy's eye". I know I was. Then, at some point, usually when the girl is between the ages of four and nine, she is sitting on her daddy's lap, and he gets an erection. He feels guilty or embarrassed, and pushes her off his lap, never explaining why, and never letting her sit there again.

Suppressed Family Incest stands in the way of every touch and affectionate gesture received later on in our lives from our partners. It gets activated especially when people move in together, or get married. At the point, when the relationship becomes familiar and like family, physical affection becomes inhibited.

The decision the little boy made after the bath scene was, "I can't have love and attention from the one I really want—my mother." The thought later in life becomes, "I can't have love and affection from the woman I want." What happens for this boy when he grows up, is one or all of the situations mentioned as questions at the beginning of this chapter. This man will choose unavailable women, like his mother. Either they will be in other relationships, far away, or too busy at work to give him the love and attention he desires.

When her daddy throws her off his lap, the girl makes the decision, "I can't have the love, attention, and affection I want from the man I want—my father." Later in life this thought becomes, "I can't have the man I want". She will choose men that are married, too busy, or far away. Or she will choose men who are loving to her, but not sexual.

Sometimes incestuous feelings are acted out, and fathers, brothers and uncles actually have sex with their daughters, sisters and nieces. If this happens, some women decide they can't trust men, or feel guilty that the sex was acted out, or can't say "no" to what they don't want, or are afraid to be sexual beings because people they don't want might want them. They also might feel they have difficulties in establishing boundaries around sex with men. Often, incest survivors will create rape situations later in their lives.

At the other extreme, some women may feel happy that their fathers, brothers or uncles loved them enough to make love to them, and decide that they can have the men they want sexually. Many years ago in the LRT, I heard a story about a father who had five daughters. He made love to four of them. The one he didn't make love to ended up in a mental institution, because she felt unloved and unwanted by her father. The other four daughters were happily married, or in good relationships with men.

I also heard about a woman who had four brothers, and made love to all but one of them. Her only regret was that she had not made love to her fourth brother. In some cultures, fathers, brothers or uncles are the ones that introduce young girls to sex. This is accepted as supportive and nurturing, and assures the girl of having her first sexual experience be pleasurable and gentle.

What is important about acted-out incest or suppressed family incest, as well as any other experience, is discovering the personal decisions that you made as a result of the event. The acted-out incest may be part of a bigger pattern of abuse that may have even started at birth. For example, if you were cesarean, you may have decided that you were controlled, abused and manipulated by your obstetrician at birth, and men in general. Later, this same decision could be acted out in incestuous acts.

Many times mothers are sexually teasing or enticing to their sons. These sons grow up to be men who create women coming on to them, but not necessarily following through sexually. I have interviewed men who felt that when their mothers' gave them enemas as children, it was sexually abusive. Toilet training can cause a man to make decisions about women controlling and manipulating men, depending upon how it was done.

The thing to remember is, we really loved our parents when we were little. They were our idols, our movie stars to look up to, especially when we were under the age of six. This is when many of our major decisions about sexuality were made. It's a good idea to take out pictures of your parents and family when you were young, to see how physically attractive your parents really were. I have pictures of my parents in their twenties, and they were both "tens."

I have been really studying and unraveling my own personal incest case. I feel it is the major reason I haven't created exactly what I want in an intimate relationship. What I want is to be married to a man I adore and want, and who adores and wants me. This man will give me everything I want: love, sex, and money.

I feel that my father has been my ideal. He is prosperous, charismatic, good looking, athletic, loves sports, a gentleman, and a great provider, father, and husband. He and my mother have been married fifty-seven years. They are happy, and have a great relationship. The interesting thing is that all three of their daughters, myself and my two sisters, are divorced and have not remarried. At the present time, all three of us have the last name Levand. I feel that I am married to my father on some level. I have made my father out to be perfect. He has everything I want.

Because he really didn't want me as a woman, he wanted a boy and he was married to my mother, I made the decision the men who have everything I want, don't want me. I have created lots of wonderful men in my life. However, I have always made sure they were not everything I wanted, because then they wouldn't want me. Since the men I choose don't have everything I want, they want me.

Jeff is more like my father than any other man I have ever found. He is a "man's man": athletic, good looking, supportive, loving, and a gentleman. I love everything about him, except that in the past few years he hasn't been as motivated about his career and money as I have. I have wanted him to be equal, or better than me, in this area.

It was important for me to have something "off" in my relationship with Jeff, because then he would want me. Since Jeff isn't perfect like I see my dad, who I knew I couldn't have, it was OK to be with Jeff, because he would not reject me. My fear was that if he were perfect and successful at his career like my father, then he would reject me. I am now willing to have the man I want, have everything I want, and to have him want me.

Writing this book on sexuality, and teaching two LIGHTENING UP ON SEX weekends in Australia and New Zealand in one month, brought up everything for me for healing in my sexuality. Incest was what I really got a chance to look at.

I will start by sharing some insights I have had about myself in relationship to my father, grandfather, mother and grandmother, as I was growing up.

My father was the only boy in a family of four children—he had three sisters. He carried on the Levand name for my grandfather. My father has always made a big deal about carrying on the family name: this was the main reason he wanted a son. He didn't have a son, but now he has three grown daughters, ages 39 to 54, who all have the Levand name.

Three days ago was Mother's Day. On that day, I was really thinking about the whole idea of how I was married on some psychic level to my father—I even have his name. I have never let another man be everything to me, because I haven't let go of my father. All of this was subconscious, until the last few days. I told my father he should adopt my son Jarrett, and give him the family name of Levand. Then the Levand name would be carried on. Jarrett's father has disappeared; my children have not heard from him in a year, so this seemed appropriate and perfect. I told my whole family that Jarrett would now be Jarrett Levand, so that all three of the Levand girls were free to marry, and drop the Levand name. Just thinking about this gave me a great release, and now I just have to legally change his name.

In Australia, I did consultations with two women who were virgins. They were in their thirties. When we talked about this at great length, we discovered that both these women had extreme loyalty to their fathers. Their mothers had told both of them that they knew their fathers better than their mothers did. One woman was told by her father that if she ever lived with a man before she was married, he would disown her. The other woman felt on some level that if she gave herself physically to another man, her father would die. These women have extreme cases of suppressed family incest feelings, for they had never even allowed another man to get to know them intimately. It is my opinion that on some level, we all hold ourselves back from committing fully in intimate relationships, due to our love and loyalty to our parents.

As a child, from the time I was able to climb out of my crib, I always crawled into my parents' bed, in between my father and my mother. I would cuddle with them. I always wanted to be close to my father. I know this was the beginning of my incest pattern with my father. I did this up to the age of eight. I would also climb into bed with my father's father, whom I adored. I was always combing my grandfather's hair, and taking care of him. I remember pretending I was his wife. Deep down, I felt I would make a better wife for both my father and grandfather then my mother and grandmother. At least when I was three to eight I thought that, and on some level I kept that thought as I grew up.

Growing up, I never felt that close to either my mother or my grandmother. My mother and I fought all the time. I was an Aries and so was she, so we both had a lot of fire, and very little things would spark off an explosive argument between us. I remember her yelling at me all the time as a child. I would always get right back at her. When I was very young, I would run to my father for protection. My father always defended me.

However, if my dad was mad at me, my mother would defend me. I really knew how to play my parents against each other. I was an expert at getting in the middle of them, just like I would get in the middle of them in bed. I was always able to look innocent. When I was becoming an LRT trainer, I recreated this quite a bit with the other trainers. Sondra Ray would defend me or support me, and Bob Mandel or Peter Kane would be processing me. I always had someone disapproving of me and someone defending me, until I got off this dynamic. Getting off it was recognizing it and CHOOSING OUT OF THE PATTERN.

I really didn't like my mother much as I was growing up. Now I love her, and feel very supported by her. When I was growing up, I was angry at her, and resented her for having my father when I wanted him. This was not a conscious thought as a child: then I felt I didn't like her because she was too busy, and never there for me. Now, I realize I probably pushed her away a lot because I wanted my father's attention so much. I did everything to get my father's attention and love. Because I didn't really like my mother that much, I identified with my father more, and became a real tomboy, so I could get his approval in that way. I fought with my mother over everything. I feel I really fought because I was jealous of my mom for having my dad.

This may seem a bit exaggerated to you: the first time I heard about Suppressed Family Incest, I thought it was ridiculous as well. It has taken me seven years to understand this fully, both intellectually, and in my body on a cellular level. The reason I am confessing my whole case is to clear it for myself, and also to help others understand the pattern more easily and more quickly than I did.

The way I have acted out this pattern of incest in my life has been amazing. We tend to create partners like our parents, because our minds thrive on familiarity. Usually we will attract partners like the parent we had the hardest time with, in order to work out our relationship with that parent. Most of my early relationships were with people who had my mother's personality type, or treated me like my mother treated me. I also created the men I loved wanting other women sexually.

I created my first boyfriend breaking up with me every year for five years, in order to explore another woman sexually. In my marriage, I created my husband having several affairs with women that were my friends. I was always creating a third party in my relationships. This is a definite incest pattern. I was always in the middle of my parents.

After I took the LRT, this pattern became more subtle, but was still there. I created a partner who didn't have affairs with other women, but he loved porno movies and dirty magazines. He was more turned on to the movies and magazines then he was to me.

When I was thirteen, my father commuted to Chicago for one year for business. I only saw him one weekend a month, or even less sometimes. I was devastated, and really missed him. I had to be with my mom full time, and learn how to get along with her. My father finally came back when my mother got cancer of the eye. He never commuted again. He then got started in the real estate business in Beverly Hills. Often, he would take me with him if he had famous clients. I remember showing houses to the Smothers Brothers, and Elizabeth Taylor and Eddie Fisher. The decision I made about the time my father was in Chicago was, 'The men I love leave me, or they live a long distance away.'

Once I healed my relationship with my mother, which I did through forgiveness, I finally created someone who I felt was like my father. He was the first man like my father I had ever dated. He looked like him a bit, did well financially, and I saw a lot of my father's characteristics in him. Since I set him up to be my father, he also acted out for me some of the negative decisions I had made about my father. As soon as I started dating him, he started traveling to Chicago on a fairly regular basis. He had never been to Chicago till he met me. He would call me from Chicago, and kid me about being like my father. We dated a couple of months, and he was constantly travelling, just like my father. The men I love are too busy with work to be there for me. He went to Africa for four months. When he came back, he broke up with me, never explaining the reason. Several months later, he confessed to me that he had a relationship with another woman when he was away that made him realize he didn't really want me.

I also had several long-distance relationships with men I had met in Greece and Sri Lanka. These were also manifestations of this incestuous relationship I had with my father.

Jeff and I have been together for the last two years. I have sold my house and am leaving Los Angeles in one month. This has put a strain on our relationship, because Jeff is an actor, and wants to continue living in Los Angeles, in order to focus on his acting career for at least the next six months. I have again set up a possible long-distance relationship. I started feeling like Jeff didn't want me. I also felt impatient that I wasn't getting everything I wanted in the relationship, even though I had set it up that way. Sex had really diminished, in terms of how much we were making love, in the last several months. I stuffed my feelings, and didn't communicate what I was feeling. The result was that I gained about ten pounds. Even when I ate less, I still kept gaining weight because I was stuffing my feelings.

Before I went to Australia and New Zealand for a month of work, I had an astrological reading for the upcoming six months with a wonderful psychic astrologer. He told me I was going to meet someone in Australia who would intrigue me, and make me seriously question what was off in my relationship with Jeff.

The main thing I became aware of was how I had stuffed my feelings, and not asked for what I wanted. I didn't ask for what I wanted because I felt I didn't deserve it. The man I met in Australia was young, very alive, very motivated to make money, had a great body, and loved music and dancing. We really got to act out our incest cases to the hilt. I was the same age as his mother. He was unwanted and illegitimate, and his parents had tried to abort him. He was addicted to chasing women who were not available, and didn't want him.

Once I surrendered and let him want me, he rejected me and didn't want me as a woman, just like my dad. We played out this scenario for seventeen days, going back and forth between being wanted, being unwanted, and rejecting each other. The main thing I learned was about my incest pattern, and about my addictions to being unwanted as a woman, and to feeling I didn't deserve what I wanted.

Being in Australia and so far away from home, I felt like I was on a different planet from Jeff. I felt as though I was sucked into a "black hole" of acting out both our cases. The man I met in Australia had also dated a very good friend of mine, who often feels like my sister on some level. I saw very clearly all four of our movies acted out before my eyes. It was really the classical incest dynamic. All four of us, on some level, were unwanted, or wanted for the wrong reasons.

I could see the addiction, and the excitement there was in not being wanted. I had Jeff, who wanted me, but didn't have everything I wanted. This fit in with his thought that he was wanted for the wrong reasons. I was also questioning if he really wanted me, because he wasn't moving with me. My girlfriend had a boyfriend who wanted her, but she felt more excited about the guy I was seeing in Australia, who only wanted her when she was unavailable, or didn't want him. Their patterns were almost identical—their conception, womb, and abortion traumas matched up perfectly. They were really turned on and excited about their dynamic. Jeff had been betrayed by every best friend he had ever had, and since I was his best friend, I had to betray him in order to honor his thoughts.

I also realized how angry I was at men for all the past hurt I had had. I really wanted to get even with men. In the LRT I was leading in Sydney, Australia, I created having the person who was ironing my clothes burn a hole in the white outfit I wear for the God section of the Training. I knew from that result that I was burning up with anger. I had stuffed all my feelings about Jeff, and my anger at men. It all came up to the surface in order to be healed.

When I left Australia I felt my love and appreciation for Jeff a lot. It was my intention to clear everything with him, tell the truth, and get what we both wanted. What we both wanted was love, prosperity and sexual bliss. Since I have been home, we are moving through all these issues.

I knew that I had a lot to work out with my father. For three years, I worked with him as Vice President of his steel business, and as a real estate salesperson under his broker's license. This gave me an opportunity to be with him a lot, which is what I initially wanted. It also gave me the opportunity to tear him down from the pedestal I had placed him on. I saw his disapproval, and his imperfections. I love him for all of his imperfections, but I don't have to idolize him.

This month, I am letting go of my father by letting go of and moving from my home of six years, for which he is the mortgage co-signer. I feel I am finally divorcing my father. The first step to getting through an incest pattern is recognizing you have it. Sometimes, we recognize we have a pattern by seeing the results in our lives. Then we can trace back the results to the earlier decisions. Whenever a pattern comes up very strongly, like this incest pattern did for me, it is ready to be released. What is up is on the way out. Thank you, God.

By looking at the questions I asked at the beginning of this chapter, you can take a look at the results you have in your life in relationship to the incest pattern.

Take some time to look at your past, and what you have created in your intimate relationships. Do the following exercises.

1. When and with whom have you been rejected in a relationship, without knowing why?
2. When and with whom have you been attracted to someone who is not available, or married?
3. When and with whom have you been involved with someone who was not available, or married?
4. When and with whom have you had a relationship where you or your partner have pulled in a third person?
5. When and with whom have you had a long-distance relationship?
6. When and with whom have you had a relationship where your partner seems unavailable, because work or a hobby seems more important to them than the relationship?
7. When and with whom have you had the sexual aspect of your relationship disintegrate or go flat?
8. When and with whom have you had a relationship in which, when you moved in together, one or both of you were no longer interested in sex?
9. When and with whom have you had a relationship where during pregnancy, or after having a child, or when it felt like family, you and your partner stopped being turned on?

If you notice, after doing the following process that you have an incest pattern, congratulations! The first step in releasing this pattern is recognizing it. The next step is to admit your addiction to the pattern. The third step is saying "no" to all unavailable men or women, and long-distance relationships.

Telling the truth and communicating is very important. When you feel really stuck in the pattern, you can get rebirthed, or have a couples consultation with someone you trust.

If your relationship gets stuck sexually after moving in together, buy some sexy clothes, go on dates, take mini-honeymoons to new and exciting places regularly. It's nice to go away to a new place every other weekend. This helps to keep a relationship fresh. Go on dates and passionately make out, and don't have sex for about a week. Keep the relationship young and alive.

It doesn't work not to tell the truth and resent your partner; you could get fat like me. Go for solution and get support.

Suggestions for Getting Through the Incest Pattern

1. The Forgiveness Diet is powerful and very releasing. It was created by Sondra Ray. Forgiveness is the "Master Erase"—it releases you from the burdens of the past. To do the Diet, you write, "I forgive myself completely." You write this seventy times each day, for seven days. Midweek, you write seventy reasons why you forgive yourself. It's OK to repeat reasons if you can't think of seventy.

1ST WEEK: I forgive myself completely. (70 x 7)

MIDWEEK: I forgive myself completely for wanting my father.

2ND WEEK: I forgive my father completely. (70 x 7)

MIDWEEK: I forgive my father completely for not wanting me as a woman.

3RD WEEK: I forgive my mother completely. (70 x 7)

MIDWEEK: I forgive my mother completely for having my father.

4TH WEEK: I forgive Jeff completely. (70 x 7)

MIDWEEK: I forgive Jeff completely for not being completely like my father.

2. Release things in your life that relate to your parents: houses, possessions, clothes, etc . . . . CLEAN HOUSE, RELEASE AND LET GO, MAKE WAY FOR THE NEW!

3. Make up a fantasy story on how you would have liked it to be, in terms of love, affection and sex with your parents.

4. Write a description of your ideal sexual experience, asking for everything your want. Describe where and how you want to be touched or kissed. What positions you haven't tried, and would like to, and your favorite positions. Describe a sexual fantasy you could do with your partner. Then write down all your fears of communicating this to your partner. Share your fears of communicating what you want to your partner, then share everything you wrote, and then act it out.

5. If you remember when affection was cut off by your parents, imagine it happening differently. For example, have your parent explain to your inner child how they were feeling at the time they cut off their affection for you, and didn't say why. Have the parent tell your inner child that it's NOT THAT THEY DIDN'T LOVE YOU, IT'S JUST THAT THEY FELT UNCOMFORTABLE OR EMBARRASSED FOR FEELING SEXUALLY AROUSED.

6. If you had siblings who you were attracted to, it helps to tell them the truth and clear the energy. When I first got in touch with my incest pattern with my father, I broke out in a hot red rash. Many times, when people tell the truth about their incest pattern with their siblings or parent, they have experienced this rash.

Do some of the following affirmations on incest, in order to change the wrong thinking you had in this area.

1. Since I, ________, know I am wanted as a man (woman), I know the woman (man) I want, wants me.

2. The closer I, ________, get to my partner, the more intimate and sexual I feel, and the more intimate and sexual I feel, the closer I am to my partner.

3. I know what I want in relationships, and I know I can have it all.

4. I love my partner and myself unconditionally.

5. The more I, ________, let go of my father (mother), the more I get what I want in relationships.

6. I, ________, am now willing for my partner to surpass my father (mother).

7. I, ________, can have the man (woman) I want in a relationship be available for me.
8. It's safe for me to have everything I want with one man (woman).
9. I am just right for the man (woman) I want.
10. The man (woman) I, ________, want, who has everything I want, wants me.
11. The perfect man (woman) is available for me to have a relationship with.
12. Since my father (mother) loves and wants me, I can have the man (woman) I want.
13. I, ________, can now have love, sex, and money from one man (woman).
14. I, ________, can have sexual feelings towards my mother (father), without acting them out.
15. It's OK for me to act out my sexual fantasies about my parents with my partner instead.
16. If I, ________, have acted out incest, I am innocent, and I can forgive myself even if I enjoyed it, and whether or not I initiated it.
17. I trust myself not to commit acts of incest, even though I did in the past.
18. It's OK to be attracted to my father (mother); I don't have to make love to my mother (father).
19. I am now willing to experience the incestuous feelings I have toward my mother, father, brother, sister, or children.
20. I forgive myself for wanting to make love to my father (mother).
21. I forgive my father (mother) for not making love to me.
22. I forgive my mother (father) for having my father (mother).
23. I forgive myself for being in the middle of my father and mother.
24. I forgive myself for having more loyalty to my father (mother) than to my partner.
25. I forgive myself for creating incestuous relationships.

26. I forgive myself for feeling I don't deserve the relationship I want.

27. I deserve to have the relationship I want.

If the appropriate affirmations are not listed, practice creating your own affirmations, tailor-made for you.

Sexual Jealousy

When we are in an intimate relationship, we often think of our partner as our possession. If someone else wants the attention of our partner, or if our partner gives someone else attention, we become jealous.

Jealousy usually happens when we feel or see our partner giving attention to someone other than ourselves. The attention doesn't even have to be sexual: if we have sex with our partner, we often feel that they belong exclusively to us.

Jealousy is the result of the thoughts that there is a scarcity of love, or there is not enough love, and that the source of love is outside ourselves. Jealousy in the present, is the result of unresolved rage from the past. This rage comes from feeling that we did not get all the love and attention that we wanted from our parents. Usually jealousy is the result of unresolved incest patterns, or sibling rivalry issues. In both cases, we were longing for the attention of one or both of our parents.

In the incest pattern, we were competing with our mother or father for the parent of the opposite sex. Gay people possibly were competing for the parent of the same sex. Either way we lost out, and the result was that someone else, our mother or father, got the love and attention we wanted. Later on, in our intimate relationships, we create triangles, or pull in a third party, in order to re-create the jealousy from our childhood that we never healed.

Usually we are very unconscious about this, and do not remember being jealous of our parent. I remember not liking my mother very much as I was growing up. I used to feel it was because we yelled at each other, she seemed angry and impatient with me and my friends, and she always complained about taking me places I wanted to go. The truth was that I didn't like my mother because she had my father. I made up reasons not to like her that seemed to be real and make sense to me.

The effect this jealousy had on my intimate relationships was that I always pulled in other women to be jealous of. In my first intimate relationship, my partner and I broke up every year for five years, for about a month, so that he could be sexual with other women. In my marriage, my husband had affairs. He kept the first affair a secret from me for several years. Underneath, I knew, because I was extremely possessive and wanted to be with him every minute. I was even jealous if he went to play basketball with the boys.

The ultimate rage I had involving jealousy occurred on my birthday, nine days after my son was born. My husband was making love with my best friend. They had gone up the hill behind our house and made love. They admitted this to me when I confronted them about what I intuitively felt in my body. I went outside in a rage and climbed up the hill behind my house. I cried, screamed and threw rocks down the mountain until I felt less rage. In all my relationships, I always created someone or something to be jealous of.

In one relationship, I didn't draw in another woman, I attracted a man who loved to watch porno movies before and during making love. I became jealous of the women in the movies. I felt as though I was lacking something, and that was why he liked to watch the movies. I was jealous of the women because they always had bigger breasts than I did. They seemed to get more of my partner's attention than I did.

After taking the Loving Relationships Training several times, rebirthing, and doing the Forgiveness Diet on my mother (See chapter on forgiveness), I stopped creating jealousy situations. The better my relationship with my mother became, the less jealousy I experienced. I finally created a partner who was there for me 100%.

Then a funny twist happened. I created my partner being jealous. This was still my jealousy case. I wanted him to be jealous in order to prove that I was wanted and desirable as a woman. I still did not believe that I was completely and really wanted to the core of my being. Because I didn't know inside myself that I was wanted, I needed him to be jealous in order to prove to me that he wanted me.

If you have jealousy in your relationship, whether it's you or your partner who is jealous, it is still your jealousy case. In order to stop creating jealousy, you have to be willing to see your payoffs for having jealousy in your life. You also have to be able to own and admit your past rage and jealousy as a child, which needs to be healed.

You could also be creating jealousy because of sibling rivalry. This would be so if you had to compete with your siblings for your parents' love and affection. In this way, you could become addicted to competition and lose/lose situations. The truth is, the more my sister gets love and affection, the more love and affection I receive, and the more love and affection I receive from my parents, the more my sister receives.

Look at who you are competing with now, who you are jealous of. Who were you jealous of as a child? Do the Forgiveness Diet on the person you were jealous of as a child. If you are willing to do that, the jealousy in your life will clear up.

Most people feel jealousy from time to time. The best way to move through jealousy is to tell the truth about it; admit you have it going on. Take responsibility for creating the jealousy situation: be willing to forgive the past and let it go.

Jealousy is a "free rebirth from the universe." If you are experiencing jealousy, go to your rebirther and heal your past fear of loss, and your rage at not receiving the love and affection you desired.

Jealousy is one of the most uncomfortable feelings I have ever experienced. I am sure everyone will agree they would rather do without it in their lives. It comes from low self-esteem, but it takes high self-esteem to tell the truth about jealousy, admit to the feelings, and be willing to let them go. The more you realize you are good enough, wanted, lovable, that there is more than enough love to go around, and that you are the source of love in your life, you will experience jealousy less and less, and experience bliss more and more. Feeling jealous offers a good opportunity to jump to a higher level of loving and appreciating yourself.

Once I understood what jealousy was all about and took steps to heal it, I released the old pain and rage. I no longer needed to create it in my life, either as a jealous person, or as someone trying to make my partner jealous, to prove to myself that I was lovable. With jealousy out of the way, sex is easier, more fun, and used less as a tool for manipulation.

Written Processes for Jealousy

1. As a child I was jealous of ________.
2. People I have been jealous of in my intimate relationships are ________.
3. List all the times you have felt jealous in your intimate relationships.
4. My payoffs for having jealousy in my life are ________.
5. My fears of giving up jealousy are ________.
6. I am now willing to forgive myself for being jealous of ________.
7. I now forgive myself for creating jealousy situations with ________.
8. I now forgive ________, because I was jealous of him (her).

Affirmations for Jealousy

1. I love myself enough to never be jealous again.
2. I am happy that my parents love each other. I can now have my own relationship with a man (woman), without jealousy.
3. I am now willing to release all jealousy from my past.
4. It's easy to tell the truth about my jealousy.
5. The more I love myself, the less jealousy I experience.
6. It's easy to let go of my jealousy.
7. The more I love myself, the more I trust my partner.
8. The more I trust my partner, the less jealousy I experience.
9. There is an abundance of love in the universe for me.
10. I am the source of abundant love in my life.
11. I no longer need my partner to be jealous in order for me to know I am loved.
12. It's safe to let go of jealousy, and experience deeper levels of intimacy.
13. I love myself whether I am jealous or not.

Help Me in Sex

The helplessness pattern is one that says "I can't," or "I don't know." Sometimes, in sex, we pretend that we're helpless and say "I can't," and "I don't know how to do it."

The helplessness pattern begins at birth, when the person feels either that they can't make it, or they're stuck, or they need help. An adult with this pattern creates partners to take care of him or her.

People who were induced, or had lots of drugs, or forceps or cesareans, may feel helpless in initiating sex. Once they get started, they love sex. The helplessness just comes in about initiating sex, because they felt they needed help at their birth.

People stuck in the helplessness pattern are stuck in their infancy. They want a partner to take care of them; they want to be nurtured and loved by their partner. They pretend they can't manage, so that they can feel helpless like they did as infants. This is especially true for people who felt they didn't really get all the love, touching and nurturing they needed in infancy.

Sometimes people use helplessness to control their partners. Getting sick is a way to be helpless and taken care of. Often this works too well. People get taken care of, but then they are helpless to get better. "I can't", or helplessness, is a way of giving up your power. Some people indulge in "I can't" so much, they actually die.

The way to get through helplessness is to really indulge in it. Have your partner or friend give you a Helpless Day, when they completely take care of everything you want and need.

If you are into control, you could also be resisting being helpless. Taking a Helpless Day helps to let go of the control. You also could learn to receive a lot of sexual pleasure from your partner. You could have a Helpless Day, and ask your partner for everything you always wanted sexually. Something fun to do is to have your partner bathe you. This is a very sensuous experience, which allows you to really surrender to your partner.

People who feel helpless might feel as though they don't know what they want sexually. They feel helpless about knowing what they want, as well as feeling helpless about receiving what they want. You do know what you want sexually. It's safe to ask for it, and you deserve to receive it.

Affirmations

1. I can have what I want sexually.
2. I know what I want sexually.
3. I can initiate sex.
4. I know how to initiate sex.
5. It's safe to let go of control in sex.
6. Letting go of control in sex gives me what I want.
7. It's safe to be loved, nurtured, and touched by my partner, without feeling helpless.

8. I can take care of myself, and it's OK to let my partner take care of me sexually.

The Struggle with Sex

Many people have a real struggle with sexuality. We talk about the Struggle Pattern in the LRT. People are used to the struggle they had at their birth and with their parents, so they continue to struggle in their intimate sexual relationships.

I had a forty-eight hour labor, and it was a bit of a struggle to get out. My sex life used to be a big struggle. I used to struggle to have sex, struggle to enjoy sex, struggle to have an orgasm, and struggle to please my partner. All the struggle didn't leave me any room for fun and pleasure.

I even struggled to heal my sexuality. I tried hard to get it right. The words that go along with struggle are "I have to". I felt that I had to get sex right, as if my life depended on it. The truth is, the more we relax and let go, the easier sex and pleasure become. The affirmation for struggle is, "If it is easy for me, it is right for me."

The struggle at our birth occurred either because we were holding back, or our mothers were holding us back, perhaps because they didn't want us, or were afraid, or both. First babies usually have more struggle than later babies. This is because mothers who have had one child know what to expect, and can relax. I was holding back when I was born, because I knew I was the wrong sex.

My mother was holding back because she had some anxiety about having a new baby to take care of. Having a baby meant a loss of independence for her. She had two children, ten and fourteen years old, and had gotten through that period of having to really be there for a baby a long time before. Letting go, for my mother, meant giving up control and independence. Consequently, in my own sexuality, it took me a long time to learn to relax and let go.

I started to let go and relax more in sex after I had my two children. With my first child, Raynbow, I had a four-hour labor. Jarrett had a forty-five minute labor. The second one was easy, and I discovered how easy and pleasurable it was to let go.

Let go of the struggle with your sex life, and just start having fun with your partner. The more ease you feel, the more turned on you will be with your partner.

Struggle occurs when you try to make something happen, instead of just allowing something to happen. The harder you try, the worse it gets. Give up, surrender, and have fun. Then sex will be easy and pleasurable.

Affirmations

1. When sex is easy, it is right for me.
2. It's safe to relax and let go in sex.
3. The easier sex is, the more alive I feel.

Guilt Closes the Door to Passion

Guilt is the major feeling to heal in order to create blissful, passionate sex in your life. In the LRT, we say "guilt demands punishment." If there is guilt, it is impossible to feel innocent and have total pleasure.

Where did we get our guilt from? It almost seems as though we were born with it. Many of us made a decision right at birth, and sometimes even before birth, that we were guilty. This is called the Infant Guilt Syndrome. Because our mothers had pain, or had drugs to eliminate pain at our births, we made the decision that our aliveness or our presence created pain for our mothers. The more pain or struggle our mothers had, the more guilt we felt. We took responsibility for our mothers' pain, and became guilty and fearful that we would always hurt the one we loved.

If your mother died, or almost died, while giving birth, your guilt could be overwhelming. The more pain associated with the birth, the more guilt you feel. The result in later life is that you feel you have to hold back your aliveness in order to protect your partners, the ones you love. You stop your energy and aliveness in order not to hurt your partner, so you don't have to feel even more guilt. When you feel like this, you are afraid to be truly intimate out of fear of being hurt or hurting your partner.

You could also feel guilty about your conception. If your parents didn't want you, you were a mistake, or they wanted the opposite sex, you could feel extreme guilt for deciding to come when you were not wanted. Then you make two major decisions: "I am unwanted" and "I am guilty for being unwanted."

You could feel guilty the whole time you are in the womb, either for not being wanted, or for being the wrong sex. If your mother had morning sickness and nausea, you could decide, "I am the cause of my mother being sick and uncomfortable."

If your parents were disappointed at what sex you were, you could feel guilty for causing them disappointment.

We also have guilt handed down from generation to generation. There is "Jewish guilt," "Catholic guilt," and "Christian guilt." We are not only guilty for our survival and our being, we also feel sinful if we are sexually alive beings. We are told by our churches, temples, parents, nuns, rabbis, ministers, and priests that sex for pleasure, especially before marriage, is a sin. Also we are told that it's not okay to touch yourself and have pleasurable sexual feelings.

All of us have sexual feelings as infants, when we are cuddled, stroked, and tickled. As four-year-olds, we have sexual feelings, just as we do in puberty. We feel a lot of sexual excitement in our bodies at these times, and because we are told by outside sources that this is not okay, we immediately feel guilty for our excitement and sexuality. The people that tell us it isn't okay were also told it was not okay, and these beliefs are passed down from generation to generation.

It's time to tell yourself it's okay to be a sexual being, that you're innocent for being a sexual being and having sexual feelings in your body. It's normal and natural to have sexual feelings and energy. Everyone has these feelings. The more guilt you have, the more you stuff these feelings and try to hold the sexual energy back. This usually creates pain in your body, or really holds you back from being creative in your life. Also, you can inhibit the flow of money in your life by holding back your sexual energy. And when you hold back your sexual energy, you become angry and resentful, especially toward anyone who you think made you feel guilty.

Besides creating pain in your body, anger and resentment anesthetize your body, and keep you from feeling the total pleasure that is your divine right.

Many of us also bought into the Adam and Eve scenario that we were thrown out of the Garden of Eden. Women unconsciously choose to feel guilty for eating the apple. Eating the apple was choosing to be separate from God, and not knowing you are at one with God. This is the place where many of us saw ourselves as separate from God instead of at one with God, and we have felt guilty for this decision ever since. This guilt has created lots of punishment, in all the wars we have fought over the centuries in the name of religion. It has been the basis for one religion saying it is better than another.

We are innocent. We are part of God: we are God. "God's will for us is perfect happiness." (Lesson 101 in *A Course in Miracles*). Anything that makes us joyous and happy is innocent for us and everyone else. Since sex is pleasurable and joyous, it is right and innocent for us.

Guilt is also the decision we make that mainly causes diseases in our bodies. When you are guilty about sex, you can end up with AIDS, prostate cancer, cancer of the female sexual organs, herpes, vaginal infections, and bladder infections. Remember that "guilt demands punishment," so the more guilty you feel about your sexuality, the more intense the punishment you will receive. The biggest forms of punishment we are creating now are AIDS and cancer.

Many men I have interviewed who have AIDS have admitted that they feel extreme guilt, and have the fear that they hurt women. They really think they hurt their mothers. They unconsciously avoid being with women in order to avoid hurting them. When they are with men they still feel guilty, so they end up punishing themselves with AIDS.

Many men with AIDS have also told me that they feel so guilty, they feel they don't deserve to be here. They feel they deserve to die. These are just wrong decisions about themselves; the truth is that they are totally innocent.

Here is the story of a gay man from New Zealand and how his birth, conception, and Personal Lie affected his sexuality.

"I was unplanned and unwanted. My mother was in her mid-forties when I was conceived. My parents already had five teenagers. My mother felt a great deal of sexual guilt in front of her five teenagers about being pregnant at her age. She felt too old to have a child: her health was bad, and she felt she would die in childbirth. She hated being seen pregnant, and felt embarrassed with doctors, in the hospital, and in public. I was born fast, with forceps and anesthesia and loaded with guilt I'd received from my mother. This guilt was all I knew, so I went through life manifesting more and more of it, as if I needed guilt to survive.

"I was sexually molested by men several times when I was three and four. I had a strict Catholic upbringing. At thirteen, I had a great deal of guilt because I knew I was gay. I could never come to terms with my sexuality. I needed loads of alcohol and drugs to have sex, because of the guilt and the anesthesia I had had at birth. Because of the forceps, I found it hard to let go, and I disliked being touched and manipulated. I always had to be in control. My Personal Lie is that I AM UNWANTED AND UNLOVED. The kinds of lovers I attracted did not want or love me. My life wasn't very pleasant, and I was unconscious and out of my body a lot. I used drugs and alcohol to aid me in staying pretty unconscious and numbed.

"In 1986, the sexual guilt manifested in me in the form of the AIDS virus. I came up positive in a blood test, and soon developed all the symptoms of the virus. I was too sick to work, and very scared. I needed to start healing fast. A turnabout came very quickly for me when I started rebirthing. The physical symptoms vanished, and I was left with the underlying causes.

"With more rebirthing and the LRT trainings, I was able to become aware of my 'case' and start to move through it. I started to have real relationships and beautiful sex. Today, April 1988, I feel the AIDS virus was the best thing that ever happened to me. It was like a fast, full, speed trip to enlightenment.

All my cases came up, and I had to process them or die. I soon got rid of my death urge. I feel the AIDS virus is a wonderful healing for the planet. People infected with it can move their case quite easily if they want to, with a good rebirther. Otherwise it might take lifetimes. Today I'm still not totally off my case, but I am aware of it and still in my body trying."

This man did a four-month Synergetic Vision Program with Yve and Vince Betar in Australia. He was moving through his fear of speaking in front of groups, with the purpose of inspiring other people with his story. He no longer has the symptoms of the virus and looks very healthy. He had the commitment to reach for life and let go of his death urge. I acknowledge him for his willingness to go for it in his own life, and to be an inspiration to others.

As I said earlier, the extreme result of guilt can be death. Several years ago, I had a client who was dying of cancer of her sexual organs. She had been fighting this cancer for eight years. When I started rebirthing her, she had been told she only had two months to live. Rebirthing was her last resort. She had been seeing several therapists and a hypnotherapist. During the eight years, she had learned from Silva Mind Control how to use her mind to fight the cancer.

She was trying to do everything to heal her "incurable disease." Her main beliefs throughout her life had been that she was guilty, and that her sexuality was bad.

She was born into a Catholic family with an alcoholic father. She had recurring dreams of her father sexually molesting her, but she had no concrete memories. Her extreme hatred and resentment toward her father was eating her body away through cancer.

When she was eighteen, she had become a nun in order to escape her guilt and her father. She was a nun for eighteen years. She left the convent after having an affair with a priest, which intensified the guilt she had been running away from. After leaving, she had an eight-year relationship with a woman. During this time she was fighting the cancer in her body.

Bob Mandel says that guilt is the "mafia of the mind." Guilt always creates pain and punishment for ourselves or the ones we love. The only way to release guilt is to affirm your innocence, let go of the anger, and release the desire for revenge behind the anger. Some people get even by being sick and dying. In order to release the anger and desire for revenge, we have to move into forgiveness. Forgiveness is the "master erase" says the *Course in Miracles*. Forgiveness is the most direct route to heal guilt, anger and the desire for revenge. The Course says that "Forgiveness is selective remembering." This means releasing the pain and hurt of past relationships, and remembering only the love and good.

Below is a letter which my client with cancer wrote to her father. She wrote this letter in order to let go of the anger, resentment and guilt that she had suppressed all her life. This anger, guilt, and resentment were killing her. She needed to release them in order either to live, or die in peace.

November 28, 1986

Dear Dad,

By now you are pretty aware that I am writing you a letter. I want you to understand how I came to write this and why.

As you know, by medical standards, the cancer I have been fighting since 1980 is incurable. I have had to seek "alternative means" to healing: "natural" or "spiritual" means. I have been in therapy with three separate therapists, and undergoing spiritual counseling. The spiritual means for dying well, and living well or getting healed, are the same.

It is not my intent or desire to punish or hurt you—my only desire is to find the truth, tell the truth, get rid of the emotional power that has made me ill, and let it go in forgiveness.

The atmosphere in which I grew up was an alcoholic home—even if you had not been at the peak of your drinking in my emotional past, I learned one lesson very well. Take care of mom and dad emotionally—my emotions come second or last.

To this day I still have a very difficult time being with you or mom, as I feel you often as an "emotional vampire"—that the very life is being drained out of me. As I became a teenager you yelled at us until we cried tears for you, so that you would know you "got to" us. That continued into my twenties. I sometimes felt that you needed my emotion and reaction to know that you existed. In therapy, my therapist asked me if I had ever had any recurring dreams, as we were seeking the source of my deep anger and resentment. The only recurring dreams I had were from ages eleven to fifteen, of my father approaching me in a sexual way, touching me in a sexual way, or forcing me in a sexual way. I told her they were "Just dreams." and "Doesn't everyone growing up have dreams like this?" She said no—only those who have a reason, those that have been abused in some way. I have not yet uncovered anything so specific. In deep therapy, I keep coming close to something awful around age three or four, but so far I have not found the memory. I have blocked it.

I have no intentions of making anything up that I can't specifically remember. However, there is a history of sexual impropriety, and some abuse from you through the years, and this has been a source of great anger, frustration, resentment and sometimes *rage* in me. I feel exploited and betrayed of the trust I should have had in a parent. Some of this is also a chauvinistic attitude on your part about women in general, or more specifically, that your children are here for your pleasure and your whims and needs.

I am going to try to go through these here as specifically as possible—remember that if I tell you the truth, then I am free. I can let it go—what you do with this information is up to you. I can't protect you from it.

You would never keep the confidence I placed in you. If you thought it would make you look good, you'd tell anything told to you in confidence. Mom is the same way. I remember telling you I wanted to join the convent. I asked you not to tell anything to anyone, only to come home to hear you blasting it all over the place to your friends. You felt I was your captive because I was your child—you did not need to respect me. That hurt.

When we differed in opinion, you, like a bully, shut me down, called me stupid, or slapped me in the face if you felt my frustration was "disrespectful" to you. You never felt you had to respect me. On the one hand, you admired my intelligence, and on the other, you denied it and tried to make me smaller—just like you made mom smaller—less than you, to make yourself bigger, important and have everyone look to you.

I was a finalist in the California scholarship and you refused to file the papers—so that I lost the scholarship. Your reason was that you were not letting me go to the convent. You wanted me to be in the business world, and "girls don't need an education" and "let the nuns pay for it." I was crushed and enraged but had to "stuff it."

You love to talk to me as though I am irresponsible and squander money. Four major surgeries in six years would make it difficult for anyone, plus eighteen years in the convent does not make a good credit record. You love to put me down, and when I was down you pushed me down further, while telling me "I want to be closer to you." It makes me feel, "What's the use? All my father does is play power games."

Come off it, Dad. You are still an adolescent acting like you don't want anyone telling you what to do. Time to grow up and put that behind you and be a man. The loving man you were meant to be, not the lecherous, grabby, selfish, grouchy, insulting drunk I see before me. Where is your dignity? And give me mine!

You didn't even allow my sisters and me the choice as to whether or not we sat on your lap or kissed you "on the lips." I didn't trust you, and you forced the issue. Do you know how that makes me feel about you? So many years, and even today I don't feel safe and respected in your love. "Kiss me, you sexy wench," you say to me. Or more recently, when I called to tell you my operation was going to be on November 7, you said "You know what would make me happy? Honey, move to another town where no one knows you, and go to a motel and find some nice man, and screw him and screw him and screw him, then you'd be okay. *Is this the talk from a father to a daughter? I am your daughter—respect me as such.*

You belittle those I love, and at the same time you want me to love the ones you love and hate the ones you hate. I am not your extension. I am a person in my own right. I am a free woman, free from you, and I will choose my life. You have always been prying, invasive, and disrespectful to me, your daughter, insisting on spanking me "with pants down" after puberty. Do you know how deeply humiliating and abusive that was?

All you want is for us to tell you the good things, like how wonderful you are. But if you don't know the truth, how can you make amends and recover? How am I to recover if you have never heard my feelings? You have ignored my thoughts and feelings, minimized them, even made fun of them because I was so threatening. I need to tell you this and I am setting myself free.

And what about all those lurid tales of sex, rape, prostitution, and white slavery you always told. Do you think that inspires a young woman to dream of taking a lover to bed? I had bad dreams for years over it. It wasn't the stories so much, as the great pleasure you took at my consternation, my discomfort. Dad, you have been sexually attracted to me for some time. I am not the one to satisfy your desire for vicarious pleasure. You have thought of me as naked in bed with my legs spread many times. I know because you have used that image when talking to me. For example, when telling me that as a woman I would not get anywhere in business unless I learned to "lay down and spread 'em."

Time to tell the truth, time to clean up your act. At every turn of womanhood when I was growing up, you were ominously there. Instead of "You're beautiful, I am proud you are my daughter." I would have to listen to "You look pretty desirable, or sexy, or look at those bumps in front." Also, you made remarks about my bras. I used to put them in the middle of a stack of clothes so I wouldn't have to listen to your remarks. Constant remarks about my period, sanitary napkins, etc., never being discreet, always long-winded and in front of anyone and everyone.

I am a woman who challenges you, thinks well, and has a will of her own. I am not mom or like mom for you. You can not run me over anymore. I refuse to leave my dignity outside the door when I see you. I won't shut up, and I won't stop telling the truth. You only pretended that the truth was your friend. You lie so much. If you can't accept reality, you just lie and say it isn't so. *The whole family* knows what a liar you are, and what a shit you have been to me and my brothers and sisters, making my sister and I kiss your creepy friends when they were drunk.

You may think a woman is only good for one thing—well, this woman has many things she is good for, and will not carry this baggage of pain, indignation, guilt, shame, fear, hostility, anger, and loneliness anymore. I deserve more, and I am getting more out of life than what you allow.

You feel jealousy about my friends, teacher, lover; anyone in my life who I love more than you. You are bitter that they all treat me better than you did or do. I have people who actually love me. I wonder if you ever knew what love was—always asking personal questions, and then criticizing the answer which you had no right to in the first place.

Everyone else is your scapegoat, so you will not have to face who you have become or what you have done. "You know what would make me happy?" you say. I don't care. Do you even have the tiniest idea what would make me happy? I was away in the convent for eighteen years—blessed freedom from you. You even found ways to make that wrong.

> You like to tell stories in public and shame your children. Does that give you pleasure, Dad? It must, because you do it all the time. All the neighbors were over, I was there, and you started in about when you gave us enemas as children. More specifically, when you gave ME one, because I was present. I left the group with a friend and went to the bathroom and threw up. Do you think as your children we have to put up with this crap?
>
> You also have a funny idea of success and failure in your kids. If we do well, of course it is because of you. If we don't do well, you like that more because you can feel superior and think you knew all along we'd fail. How would you react to this abuse, Dad? If I have gotten anywhere, it is in spite of you rather than because of you. You have been the biggest handicap in my life to overcome. You have been much too important to me. That has to change, because it will kill me. Do what you want with this information. Remember, please, that my purpose is healing myself. I want to forgive you. There are many decisions I have made based on these situations.
>
> As long as you see me in anything but a positive, supportive light, our relationship cannot be healed. I love you. I want to forgive and be healed.
>
> —*Your daughter*

This letter contained a lot of anger and blame, but it was the best she could do at that time. Normally, we recommend that people continue to rewrite these letters until they clear all their negative feelings, and to get to the point where they would feel good if they received the letter. Between November 28, 1986, when it was written, till February, 1987, when she died, she continued to work on healing her relationship with her father. She was determined that they would get to a place of unconditional love and approval with each other.

About a week before she died, Patrick Collard, a friend of mine and exceptional healer, worked on her in the hospital. He discovered the place in her body, in her upper thigh, that held her guilt from when she was four years old. He told me that her father had never molested her, but had fondled her when he was drinking, and she was sitting on his lap. The father had felt extreme guilt, which she had picked up and kept for the rest of her life.

Patrick never told her this, but two days later she was receiving a massage on her upper thigh and she got the exact memory of this incident. It was just as Patrick had said. She and her father were able to love and forgive each other before she died. It was as though she was waiting to receive her innocence, and give her father back his, before she died. Forgiveness gave her the ability to let go and have the peace she wanted. At that moment of peace and innocence, she knew that she could leave the body that no longer was serving her. She consciously stopped breathing, and gave up the struggle and hatred she had fought to live with all of her life.

Affirmations for Releasing Guilt

1. I am innocent.
2. My sexuality is innocent.
3. I am innocent for choosing my parents.
4. I am innocent for coming before my parents were ready for me.
5. I am innocent for choosing to be a girl.
6. I am innocent for choosing to be a boy.
7. My body is innocent.
8. My sexual feelings are innocent.
9. My sexual energy is innocent.
10. My sexual preference is innocent.
11. My sexual equipment is innocent.
12. My sexual parts are innocent.
13. I am innocent for loving my mother.
14. I am innocent for loving my father.
15. I am innocent for wanting affection from my mother.
16. I am innocent for wanting affection from my father.
17. I am innocent for touching and playing with my body.
18. I am innocent for having erections when I see beautiful men or women.
19. I am innocent for having sexual thoughts.
20. I am innocent for liking porno movies.

Sexual Performance Pressure

Another way that we beat ourselves up with our Personal Lies is with sexual performance pressure. If we don't have the big "o", or we orgasm too quickly, then we can feel not good enough, or like a disappointment. We can also feel guilty, or that there is something wrong with us.

When we are orgasm-goal-oriented in sex, we miss out on joy, bliss and the beauty of being in the moment with our sexuality. When we take the pressure off ourselves and our partner in sex, then we have more fun and bliss.

I was someone who had never experienced an orgasm with a man. I had also never experienced an orgasm with myself. Eventually I started feeling safe enough to explore masturbation, and I started to have orgasms. At first, these orgasms were nothing more than a release, and not very satisfying, because I was holding myself back.

After I took the Loving Relationships Training, started rebirthing consistently, and began to love and approve of myself as a woman, I started to open up more sexually, to relax and let more sexual pleasure in.

I feel at one time I had "penis envy", and that is why I never gave myself permission to have orgasms. The more I appreciated myself as a woman, the more the quality and quantity of my orgasms improved.

The more I released my anger and resentment toward men, that I felt because they were boys instead of me, the more pleasurable my orgasms with men became. My orgasms changed from being clitoral and localized, to coming from deep within me and shaking my body. The more I relaxed, and the less pressure I placed on myself to have an orgasm, the more orgasms I had naturally, easily and with more intensity. I started enjoying sex and intimacy for its own sake. Whether or not I had an orgasm was no longer significant to me. In the past, if I didn't have an orgasm, I would feel disappointed, and feel I was a disappointment to men. I lied about having orgasms, so that the man I was with would not feel he was a disappointment, or feel pressured because I was not pleased.

I used to feel that it took too much time to please me, and that no man would be that patient. The more I realized I deserved sexual pleasure, the easier it was for me to have orgasms.

As long as you enjoy and have fun making love, it doesn't matter whether you have no orgasms, multiple orgasms, clitoral orgasms, or vaginal orgasms. The key is being in the moment with the pleasure, rather than waiting for an orgasm, or pressuring yourself to have one.

Men sometimes feel a lot of pressure to have an erection. If they concentrate on the pleasure and the pleasing, the erection usually follows. Some men I interviewed felt pressure about whether to ejaculate or not, or how long to prolong ejaculation. I feel that if you try to prevent or delay ejaculation, that this takes you out of the moment, and often separates you from your partner.

Jeff is great at pleasing me, and usually gives me lots of time. Sometimes, he has to really concentrate to do this. His technique is that he thinks about baseball plays as he is making love, so he won't orgasm. Yes, I have more pleasure, but sometimes this makes him more distant from me, as he is trying to stall his ejaculation. Sometimes, I like it better if he just is 100% there with me and relaxes into the energy.

Men and women both feel a lot of pressure around performance and orgasms. The more we heal our Personal Lie issues and our separation issues, the less pressure we place on ourselves and our partners. This will create more love, safety and pleasure.

I feel that the thought that men better save up their semen and not ejaculate, also creates performance anxiety. This thought is coming from a deathist point of view; that our semen, life urge, and vitality run out. The more we accept our immortality, the more we let go of the idea that our semen will run out. Immortality comes from the ideas that we are safe and immortal right now, and that our life is inevitable. Physical immortality gives us more safety and aliveness in our lovemaking.

In the past, death and sex have been tied together. "Le petit mort" is the French phrase for orgasm. It means "the little death." Some people feel like they are dying when they have an orgasm. Along with this idea of dying in sex, people also often hold their breath when making love. The more you breathe during sex, the more pleasure and aliveness you feel. If people are living in their death urge, they could feel that if they really let go in sex, they could die. The result would be that they hold back, and don't receive as much pleasure as they could.

The more people rebirth, the better they find their sex life becomes. The breathing lets in more pleasure. Also, rebirthing processes people's death urges, allowing them to feel safer about really letting go in sex. The more people get rebirthed, the safer they feel with their aliveness and sexual energy.

The safer and more immortal you feel, the better your sex life will be. There is no more need or desire for sexual performance pressure; the pressure is off when you accept physical immortality. There is plenty of time and energy to have an abundance of pleasure and orgasms.

Since many of our parents are dead, or have a deathist point of view, they probably did not have immortal sex. Maybe they have the thought that they are too old for sex, or that they can no longer get it up. We no longer need to be loyal to our parents in our sexuality. It is safe to surpass our parents sexually.

Affirmations

1. I deserve to have orgasms.
2. I have sexual pleasure, whether or not I have orgasms.
3. The more in the moment I am sexually, the more pleasure I have.

4. Since I am safe and immortal right now, it's safe to really let go in sex.
5. It's safe to surpass my parents sexually.
6. I move from goal-oriented sex to spontaneous, free sex.
7. I approve of myself whether I have orgasms or not.
8. I am good enough to have orgasms.
9. It's a wonderful surprise how easy it is to have orgasms.
10. The more I relax, the more orgasms I have.

Celibate Times in Relationships

Celibacy is refraining from sex. More of our lives are spent in celibacy than in being sexual. It is important to feel good about yourself whether you are sexually active or not. Celibacy should be a conscious choice you make for yourself.

Often people are celibate because they are avoiding sex and intimacy. People can use celibacy to protect themselves, in the same way they can use weight. If you are choosing celibacy, look at your reasons. Are you avoiding intimacy because of fear? Do you feel being celibate makes you more spiritual?

Many religious people are celibate. Priests and nuns, for example, are celibate because they are married to God. In some religions, celibacy is looked at as PURE and INNOCENT. I became very close to an ex-nun at one time. She had an affair with a priest. I was shocked, and thought this was unusual. She informed me that this is more common than we would expect. The result of this union, for both people, was sexual guilt.

For my friend, this guilt resulted in cancer of her sexual organs, and ultimately, death. Her completion letter to her father is included in an earlier chapter of this book. She avoided intimacy and sex by becoming a nun at eighteen. She had a terrible relationship with her father, which was based on guilt, abuse, co-dependency and denial. The causes of all this were her father's alcoholism, and how they interacted with each other. This is an extreme case of how celibacy, based on guilt and fear, can lead to unhappiness, disease and death.

I had another client who was working on releasing cancer from her body in her rebirthing sessions. She had bouts of cancer after each of her two children were born. She shared that she attracted her husband because she was a virgin, innocent and pure. Once they were married, she never really let go and felt comfortable sexually. The sex in their marriage was difficult in the beginning, and after a while diminished to almost nothing. Her husband had affairs because he was very sexual. She was the PURE ONE, the non-sexual woman, THE MADONNA he placed on a pedestal. It was not appropriate for her to be a "sexy wife."

They experienced a lot of celibacy in their marriage, but it was not their conscious choice: it was based on how she and her husband both saw her. They both wanted to keep her the "innocent virgin." Pregnancy and birth proved that she was a sexual being. Her body and her mind were not in sync. Part of the "cancer personality" relates to being in denial. This woman denied her sexuality to herself and her husband, and this denial resulted in cancer.

Both of these examples are extreme cases, but are important in order to make a point. You are a DIVINE, SEXUAL BEING. Denying your sexuality out of fear or guilt can result in disease.

Celibacy by choice can be extremely purifying and beneficial. There was a period in my life when I chose to be celibate for nine months. I had been involved in non-stop relationships since I was sixteen, and non-stop sexual relationships since I was nineteen. One relationship would end, or be ready to end, and I would get into another one. When I was becoming a LOVING RELATIONSHIPS TRAINER, it was brought to my attention that it seemed as though I was addicted to sex. It was suggested to me that I experiment with celibacy. I chose to act upon this suggestion, and I followed through with nine months of celibacy.

What I learned in this celibate period, was that I thought having sex and being sexual was a way for me to feel good enough or wanted as a woman. I needed the external validation of sex and sexual attraction with men to feel worthy as a woman. The more I loved, accepted and wanted myself as a woman, the less I needed sex to validate myself as a woman. This celibate period gave me the opportunity to love myself unconditionally, and appreciate myself as a woman.

When I started having sex again, it wasn't from need or to prove anything. Sex became more pleasurable, in the moment, and satisfying for my partner and me. Before celibacy, I was more goal and performance oriented. I tried to really show my partners how great I was sexually, so they would want and love me. After this period of celibacy, because I wanted and accepted myself as a woman, men appreciated and loved me for who I was, whether or not I was sexual with them.

Sometimes we have celibate periods in our relationships or marriages. This is not necessarily bad. For me, this is a time to see that I love myself and my partner, and my partner loves himself and me, whether we are sexual or not. If you are going through celibate periods in your relationship, it is important not to judge yourself or your partner. Let go of any blame you have for yourself or your partner.

If you aren't having sex, ask yourself why you are choosing not to have sex. Is your Suppressed Family Sexuality Pattern (incest) being activated? Have you left the passion and romance of your relationship behind? Are you too tired, or is there not enough time? Are you in a boring rut sexually? Find out why you aren't having sex, and ask yourself if you truly want it.

Resolve the issues that keep you from having sex by recognizing the patterns and causes, and then take action. Taking action could mean scheduling romantic times alone together, or taking a little trip away from home for a few days. It could mean buying some sexy lingerie, or making a special date with each other. It could mean making your partner a romantic, candlelight dinner, or watching sexy, romantic movies.

Maybe you are just feeling non-sexual. It is important to love yourself for feeling non-sexual. The most important thing is to be conscious of the reason you are choosing celibacy. If you are conscious in your choice, then you can always choose back into being sexual whenever you want.

Celibacy based on fear, guilt or unconsciousness does not serve you or your partner. Conscious celibacy can make you feel more passionate, appreciative and loving toward your partner and yourself.

Something I have found is that most couples go through periods of celibacy, or times when they are less interested in sex. Sometimes, we think we are the only ones experiencing this, and we make ourselves and our partners wrong.

For the first nine months Jeff and I were together, sex, and exploring each other sexually, was frequent and important. This period was like being in the womb: a bonding and exploring period.

We have had other periods when we haven't felt sexual at all. We might be more focused on work, or on our personal spiritual quests. It has been important for me to make the non-sexual times OK, rather than to say, "Oh God, we are not sexual now, there must be something wrong with the relationship or us." In the past, I would make the relationship, myself or my partner wrong. Now I accept these periods, and see that it is what both of us are choosing in the moment, and at any time we can choose to be very sexual again. I also look at the value we are receiving, and that makes it exciting to choose to be sexual again.

Sometimes, in these celibate periods, you can get into the Withhold, Withdraw, Resent Syndrome. For example, Sue doesn't want sex and says "no" to her partner, Joe. The next time Sue wants sex, Joe withholds it. Sue then withdraws sexually for a week, and they both end up feeling resentment. This is also the Getting Even Pattern with sex. Since Sue didn't want Joe sexually, Joe will get even by not wanting Sue when she wants him. No one wins in this situation, and both people end up feeling badly.

It's important to be able to say "no" to sex, and know that you will not lose your partner's love. Say "yes" to sex only when you really want it.

You and your partner spend more time together celibate than you do being sexual. This is especially true of couples that are living together or married. Feeling good being celibate is just as important as feeling good being sexual. Being celibate in your relationship means loving yourself just for who you are, and loving your partner just for who s/he is. Choosing to be sexual, or choosing celibate times, is equally important for having a great sexual relationship, based on high self-esteem and telling the truth faster.

Sex and Money

Sex and money are closely related. If you feel stuck in your sexuality, you might also feel stuck in creating as much money as you want.

Sexual energy, and the energy to create money, are one and the same. You might experience more prosperity, the more you have great sex. The more you enjoy sex, the more money you will receive. Sex is about receiving from your partner. Being prosperous is about receiving from the universe. As you open up your channels to receiving more sexual energy, you are also opening up your channels to receiving more energy in the form of money.

In the '40's, Napoleon Hill wrote a book called *Think And Grow Rich,* in which he interviewed five hundred millionaires. He writes about the principles they used to create their wealth. In chapter eight, he talks about the transmutation of sexual energy. He says that the same energy that attracts a partner sexually is what you use to attract money into your life. He also says that behind every millionaire there is a woman. (This was written in the '40's, when most of the millionaires were men.)

What he was saying was that these men were sexually happy and satisfied by their partners. They had their creative, receiving energies flowing, so they created great wealth. This statement could also be true, "Behind every good woman, there is a man," or better yet, "Both men and women stand equally, mutually satisfying each other sexually, and creating large fortunes of wealth and prosperity in their lives."

Men and women who are not sexually active can also transmute and use their sexual energy to create money. I have seen people who avoid relationships, but are great at creating lots of money. They use their charisma and sexual energy to attract money. They may have a fear of intimacy, but at least they don't shut down their creative energy. Some people are so afraid of their life force that they shut down their energy, and end up poor, and with no relationships.

I notice for myself that the more I am sexually satisfied, the more income I create. If I feel stuck in the area of money, making love always moves the energy, and I create more money.

Just as with sex and everything else, it is important to look at your thoughts about money. Do the following written exercise:

1. My thoughts about money:
2. My mother's thoughts about money:
3. My father's thoughts about money:
4. My thoughts about wealthy people:

You might have judgements about wealthy people which hold you back from having the wealth you desire. If you do, then if you became wealthy, you would end up judging yourself for the same reasons you now judge wealthy people. Because you don't want to disapprove of yourself, you just avoid being wealthy.

My experience of wealthy people is that the majority are very generous with their money, and that is why they keep creating more. Elvis gave $1,000 to each of twenty-five charities, each Christmas. My father was the Man Of The Year through Gateways Hospital for contributing to numerous charities. Jerry Lewis spends time and energy raising money to fight muscular dystrophy. Elizabeth Taylor spends time and money for AIDS research. The list goes on and on. People who have money, know that the way to receive more is to give and be generous. Tithing and giving seed money works to expand your income. Just as in sex, the more you give, the more you receive.

People have the same kind of limiting thoughts about money as they do about sex. Do the following quiz. Fill in the blanks with sex, intimacy, money, love, affection, time, and security, when that makes the statement true for you. You can use more than one answer in each blank.

1. I can't get enough ________.
2. I can't have ________.
3. ________ is dirty.
4. ________ isn't spiritual.

5. There is never enough ________.

6. My parents never had any ________.

7. ________ makes me crazy.

8. I never have as much ________ as I need.

9. I have to work hard to get ________.

10. ________ is not good enough.

11. The more ________ I have, the more I want.

12. I'm too tired to get ________.

13. ________ is too much work.

14. ________ takes too much time to get.

15. Everyone else has more ________ that I have.

16. I have to do something I don't like in order to get ________.

17. I have to compromise myself to get ________.

18. I say "yes", when I mean "no", to get ________.

19. You have to save ________ up.

20. It's not OK to want too much ________.

21. If I don't have ________, I get cranky.

22. ________ never lasts.

23. ________ drains me.

24. I never tell anyone how much ________ I have.

25. I can't have more ________ than my parents.

Notice how many of the above you have filled in with sex and money. Do you have the same limiting thoughts about both? Change any negative thoughts about sex and money you have. You can make your own personal sex and money affirmation tape with your personalized affirmations.

Just as with sex, your ability to make money is affected by your conception, birth and Personal Lie.

If your conception was illegitimate, you might create money illegitimately. If you were a financial burden at your conception, you might now be a financial burden to yourself or your partner. If you were unwanted, or felt not good enough, you might feel you don't deserve to have money or sex. If you feel you are wrong, or something is wrong with you, you might not be able to create money in the right way for you. If you are guilty, you might make money but lose it, because guilt demands punishment, and sabotages you, especially in your finances.

If your birth was hard and a struggle, you will probably work hard and struggle to make money. If you hurt your mother at your birth, you might hurt people through money. If you were hurt at birth, you might feel that you get hurt by money, which might make you subconsciously push money away.

Make an Eternal Law for money to clear these issues. Examples:

SINCE I KNOW I AM GOOD ENOUGH. I DESERVE TO HAVE ALL THE MONEY I WANT.

SINCE I AM WANTED, MONEY WANTS ME.

SINCE I AM A FINANCIAL GIFT, I RECEIVE LARGE GIFTS OF MONEY.

SINCE MY ALIVENESS BENEFITS ME AND EVERYONE ELSE, MY MONEY BENEFITS ME AND EVERYONE ELSE.

SINCE I AM LEGITIMATE, MAKING MONEY FOR ME IS ALWAYS LEGITIMATE.

MAKING MONEY IS FUN AND EASY.

SINCE I KNOW I AM INNOCENT, MONEY COMES TO ME EASILY, AND STAYS WITH ME.

Money issues can be one of the biggest problems a couple face in their relationship. When two people come together with their individual money issues, the issues get magnified, and can become a main problem. It is a good idea to get to know your partner's issues about money, so that you can support each other in clearing the issues, instead of having fights about them.

I remember when I was a child, the only thing my parents ever argued about was money, and this was done behind closed doors. My bedroom was connected to my parents' bathroom, and often I could hear them arguing about money. My father thought my mother spent too much money, and my mother felt that my father did not give her enough money for food, clothes, bills, etc. My father could never figure out how she spent all the money he gave her.

Since we tend to re-create our parents' patterns, I often have Jeff asking me how I managed to spend all the money I made. I tend to be like my mother, and no matter how much money I have, I spend it. Jeff can make a dollar go a long way, just like my father.

In my parents' situation, my father made the money, and my mother nurtured my father. She made sure he was well fed and sexually satisfied. As more and more women work, and make their own incomes, the roles around sex and money become more confused. The roles in the past seemed more clear-cut. It was the man's duty to support his wife, and it was the woman's role to nurture and sexually satisfy her husband. If the woman enjoyed sex, this seemed like a good exchange, but if she didn't, it could feel like a duty, and something she dreaded. As women support themselves more, sex becomes more of a choice for them—something to love and enjoy at least as much as men do. Women are now exploring sex for their own enjoyment, instead of as a way to please and satisfy men in exchange for financial security.

There should be equality in sex and money in New Age relationships. Men and women are equal in their abilities to create money and enjoy sex. As we all come more into balance with our feminine and masculine energies, at any given moment we can switch back and forth between being the givers and the receivers of both sex and money.

In the movie *Nuts*, with Barbra Streisand and Karl Malden, there is a good example of how sex and money can become confused in relationships. As a child, in the movie, Barbra had been given money by her stepfather, Karl Malden, for giving him certain sexual favors. As an adult, she became a prostitute, and received money for giving sexual favors, just as she had as a child. This is an exaggerated example of how we set up confusion around sex and money. We think, "I will do this, and then you will give me money, or provide for me". In a situation like this, the sex is not happening because the people involved want to pleasure each other. It is happening out of a sense of responsibility and duty.

It's important to clear up any need/obligate issues you and your partner have about sex and money. If you need your partner for sex or money, they end up feeling obligated to you, and ultimately will end up resenting you. You end up resenting them as well, because of your need. When you realize that you are your own source of pleasure and abundance in your life, and your partner is the source of pleasure and abundance in his or her life, you release the need/obligate dynamic. Then you can have a relationship based on equality.

Sex and Food

Sex and food are two ways that we nourish and love ourselves. Sometimes we substitute food for sex. We use eating, getting fat, and stuffing ourselves, as ways of avoiding sex.

This starts with the Undernourishment Syndrome, when as infants we do not get what we really want. We want our mother's breast, and we get a substitute—a bottle. If you were fed on a schedule, you also might have made the decision that you had to wait for what you wanted. The two thoughts or decisions made in this situation are, "I can't have what I want" and "I can't have it when I want it."

Often we substitute food for sex. When we do this, what we really want is sex, intimacy and touching, and what we get is something to eat. When we eat, we stuff down our feelings about the closeness we really want with our partners.

Do you spend more time eating with your partner, or making love with your partner? What would you rather be doing? I have noticed that if Jeff and I eat a large meal in the evening, we never have sex. After food comes sleep. This seems to be a good way to avoid the closeness, the love and the nourishment we really want through intimacy and sex.

People who didn't get nursed as infants are often confused about whether they want sex or food. They will choose the food because they got the food at birth, but not the nourishment and closeness of the breast. They never really get satisfied, because underneath their actions is the decision about not getting what they want. They eat, thinking that is what they want. Then they get upset, because what they really want is to make love.

If you are not in a relationship, you might spend a lot of time eating, in order to stuff your feelings of sadness about being alone. The more you eat, the fatter you get, which keeps you from finding a partner, because you fall into low self-esteem about being too fat. You may have so much fear of intimacy that you use eating, food and gaining weight as ways to avoid it.

Often, we have food hooked up with love. Our parents may have given us food instead of love, affection and attention. I knew as a child that I would always have a good, healthy meal. My mother loved me through feeding me well, with nutritious food and vitamins. This is the major way she loved me. She was not a person who hugged or kissed, or gave her children a lot of physical affection. Her way of loving us was to give us the best possible meals she could: great salads and well-balanced meals. Because I was rebellious, I would crave the junk food and sweets that I was never allowed at home. Now I can see that I was also starving for affection and touching.

Since our parents usually did not feel comfortable with a lot of physical affection, they loved us the best way they knew how, which was by feeding us well.

Jeff's mom was a gourmet cook, and this was how he was loved by her. To Jeff, loving meant caring for him by preparing great meals. I don't like to cook that much, but love to go out to eat, so we nourish ourselves well that way. I often feel that Jeff feels that I don't love him, because I don't cook him gourmet foods like his mother. Sometimes, I feel he withholds sex from me because he feels I withhold cooking from him.

I have been doing a master cleansing fast over the last ten days. All I take in is water, mixed with lemon juice, maple syrup and cayenne pepper. This fast has given me the opportunity to see how addicted I am to food. So much of my time is given to eating, and thinking about what I am going to eat. The fast has given me more time to focus on writing, and pleasuring myself in other ways besides food.

Are you using food as a substitute for sex, love and intimacy? If so, you might try fasting, and working on your thoughts about receiving what you really want.

Affirmations

1. I can have what I really want—sex and intimacy.
2. I can have what I really want now—sex and intimacy.
3. I can love myself with sex and intimacy, instead of with food.
4. I nourish myself with sex and intimacy.
5. I forgive myself for using food to avoid sex and intimacy.
6. I forgive myself for using food as a substitute for sex and intimacy.
7. I forgive my mother for nourishing me with food instead of with physical affection.

CHAPTER 6

Celebrating Our Sexuality

Forgiveness Opens the Door to Hot Sex

SINCE FORGIVENESS IS the "Master Erase", healing the desire for revenge is the key to getting back to our initial innocence.

A Course In Miracles (Workbook, page 391) answers the question, "What is forgiveness?"

> "Forgiveness recognizes what you thought your brother did to you has not occurred. It does not pardon sins and make them real. It sees there was no sin. He who would not forgive must judge, for he must justify his failure to forgive. But he who would forgive himself must learn to welcome truth exactly as it is."
>
> Lesson 229 states, "Love which created me is what I am. Father my thanks to you for what I am, for keeping my identity untouched and sinless, in the midst of all the thoughts of sin my foolish mind made up and thanks to you for saving me from them. Amen."
>
> Lesson 297 says, "Forgiveness is the only gift I give because it is the only gift I want and everything I give, I give myself."

What should we forgive? What does forgiveness have to do with sex? Anger, guilt and resentment anesthetize the body, not allowing us to feel and experience the total bliss and excitement we deserve. The more you forgive, the more pleasure and excitement you will feel in your body and in your life.

How do we forgive? These are the steps to forgiveness, as taught in the Loving Relationships Training.

1. You forgive yourself:

   —for feeling guilty about your aliveness.

   —for feeling that your aliveness creates pain.

   —for feeling guilty for hurting your mother.

   —for feeling that you did hurt your mother.

   —for feeling guilty for being a man.

   —for feeling guilty for being a woman.

   —for feeling guilty for your existence because they didn't want you.

These are a few things to forgive yourself for which affect your sexuality. You can probably think of more that you can relate to.

2. Forgive them—anyone you have upsets with around the issue of your sexuality.

3. Give up all claim to punishing, or the desire to get even.

4. Eventually, others forgive you.

5. Restore good harmony, as before the event.

How do you implement forgiveness? You can do a visualization process: one of my fellow LRT trainers shared with me a story about a man whom he had a hard time forgiving. He told this man not to call him for five years. In the meantime, he visualized himself at one end of a field, and the man he was angry with at the other end. Each day, he would visualize himself moving closer to this man. When he got to the place of meeting face to face in the field, the man called. The man said, "I know it isn't five years yet, but I know the anger, and the situation has been resolved," and it had.

When you give the gift of forgiveness, you receive it back. Your perception of the person changes, and you can get back into a space of unconditional love. Since anything that you have unresolved in your relationships with yourself and your family will come up for healing in your intimate relationships, it is important to get to complete forgiveness with everyone. You know when you have completely forgiven someone when "you remember only the loving thoughts you gave in the past and those that were given you." (*A Course In Miracles*)

Another way to get to forgiveness is writing completion letters. We suggest that before you start these letters, you get out all your hate and blame toward the other person. For example, you could write at the top of the paper, "The Reasons I Hate My Mother". Then write a letter of complete blame. Blame her for everything that is wrong with your life. Then, write a letter at the total other extreme, taking 100% responsibility for everything that happened in your relationship and life. A good completion letter is one that is a balance between total blame and 100% responsibility. Take responsibility for how the person you are forgiving made you feel. What did they bring up for you by their actions?

The following letter is a completion letter I wrote my ex-husband on September 15, 1987. The result was good. We got together, and he was more willing to be supportive of me and the kids in the best way he could. My money situation improved tremendously. Shortly after writing this letter, I sold my home in L.A. and made a considerable profit. Always state in the letter that the purpose of the letter is to heal your relationship. This is a powerful tool for releasing the past, and being in present time. Remember, present time is God's time, and the best time in which to have great sex.

Dear Michael,

The purpose of this letter is to clear the past, so we can both feel better about each other now.

In the work I do, we stress forgiveness and unconditional loving. I feel that all my relationships except the one with you come out of unconditional love, acceptance, and forgiveness.

The main reason I feel that I have been unable to forgive you completely, and be more unconditionally loving to you, is that I fear being vulnerable to you again. I feel in our marriage, you were my best friend. I trusted you, and I was vulnerable to being hurt by you.

Because I had low self-esteem, and did not feel good enough or right as a woman, I created proof of that in my relationship with you, and was hurt. I now know that you did not hurt me, you were just proving to me all the thoughts I unconsciously believed about myself.

Today I had a rebirth, and my rebirther suggested that I write you a completion letter about money. I was totally resistant to the idea. So, since I know what you resist, persists, I decided to write you in spite of all my resistance.

What I realized today, is that I never made it OK to receive money from you for the kids, because I didn't think I deserved it or was worthy of it. I also had the belief that I had to make it on my own financially, in order to prove that I could be as good as a man. I have never let any man give to me financially, except my father. He has been the only one I have felt safe enough with, to let help me financially.

I realized today that I want and deserve to receive money from men. So, in order to clear this money issue, I need to open the door I closed to you. I want to open up all doors to being supported financially by men and God.

I never asked for child support from you because I had the belief you would fight me, make it difficult, and it would take less energy for me to make the money on my own. I am now willing for you to contribute to the support of your children. As they get older, they need more things. Over the past few months, I have had difficulty creating all the money I need for bills, and also to be able to give them all they need and want. I have had a hard time saying "no" to the kids, and I have bent over backwards to give them everything they want and deserve: camp, clothes, school supplies, a vacation to the Bahamas, and modeling school. I want Raynbow and Jarrett to receive all the things that we both received from our parents.

You have dropped out of sight in terms of being their father. Maybe if you contribute to their life financially, you will feel more like their father, and be appreciated by them more.

I just don't want to close any more doors on receiving money from God, and you are part of God. So I am willing to let you contribute to the children's life financially if you want. By writing this letter, I know I am no longer closing any doors. Whether you decide to contribute or not does not matter, because at least I know I am letting all the doors be open to receiving financial help.

Thank you for what you contributed to my life. I am grateful for all I have learned from you. I appreciate all the places we travelled together, how we created Mudhole Place, and of course, the best gifts I received from our marriage were Raynbow and Jarrett.

I bless you and release you, and pray for your happiness. I support you in allowing someone else into your life to love and care for.

My intention in writing this letter is to allow us to support and care for each other more, and let the past go.

Love, Rhonda

In her book, *The Only Diet There Is,* Sondra Ray presented the Forgiveness Diet. As I mentioned earlier, this is great for letting go of pounds, as well as anger and resentment.

You write each affirmation seventy times a day for seven days. Jesus said, "Forgive your brother seventy times seven." This a magical release formula.

The following list are suggestions of who to do the Forgiveness Diet with.

I forgive myself completely.

I forgive my mother completely.

I forgive my father completely.

I forgive my obstetrician completely.

I forgive God completely.

I forgive my sister completely.

I forgive my brother completely.

I forgive the whole medical profession completely, especially my gynecologist.

I forgive my ex-husband completely.

I forgive my ex-wife completely.

I forgive all my past lovers completely.

I forgive the Catholic Church completely.

I forgive Judaism, the Rabbi and the Temple completely.

I forgive the priests and the nuns completely.

Forgive anyone who you felt made you feel guilty about sex. Forgive anyone you would not feel comfortable with, if they walked into the room right now. Jot down all the names and systematically go through the list. Forgiveness makes you feel lighter, more energetic, more alive, and definitely more sexy. Forgiveness allows you to feel turned on by the whole world.

Forgiveness Affirmations

1. I am now willing to release any blocks I have to forgiving ________ completely.
2. Forgiveness is easy.
3. Forgiveness is the "Master Erase".
4. Forgiveness is the way to sexual bliss and happiness.
5. Forgiveness really works.
6. Forgiveness is fun.
7. I love forgiveness.
8. The more I forgive others, the more I love myself.
9. Forgiveness is the greatest gift I give and receive.
10. It's safe to forgive myself and others completely.

Intimacy, Sex and Passion

There is a difference between having sex, fucking, making love, and intimacy. Many of us are OK with sex as long as it is not in a permanent relationship. Other people don't want sex unless they feel really close and connected to their partner. When sex and intimacy come together, true passion is created.

I like to look at intimacy as "in-to-me-see". In order to be truly intimate, you have to be willing to let your partner see you completely and to the core. You have to love yourself, and see yourself honestly enough to allow your partner to see you.

In order to be truly intimate, you have to trust. You have to trust yourself, and women and men in general, in order to let your partner see you completely.

The following written process will help you look at your level of trust:

1. The reasons I don't trust myself are ________.

2. The reasons I don't trust women are ________.

3. The reasons I don't trust men are ________.

I have done this process many times over the years. I have found that I don't trust people in general for the same reasons that I don't trust myself. You will find a common theme running through your decisions about trusting yourself, and trusting people in general. I have also noticed that the more I do this process, the more I trust myself. Recognizing my mistrust has allowed me to release it. In order to be truly intimate, you have to feel safe with yourself, and with your partner.

1. The reasons I don't feel safe in the presence of a man (woman) are ________.

2. The reasons I don't feel safe to be intimate and sexual with a man (woman) are ________.

Many of our thoughts of feeling unsafe stem from our birth and early childhood, when we felt vulnerable, small, and somewhat helpless. As we clear our birth trauma, we feel safer and safer.

Another aspect of intimacy is surrender. Many times people feel they are giving up themselves, or something they want and love, if they surrender. In order to have intimacy really work, you have to surrender to your higher self, and to the higher self of your partner. Many people completely avoid relationships because they feel they would have to give up who they are, in order to be with and please a partner. I find that the more I do what I want, and am myself, the more Jeff does what he wants, and is himself.

Intimacy is a mutual understanding of who we each are. We can be connected and together, and we can be connected and apart. I used to feel that the only way I could be connected to my partner was to be with him twenty-four hours a day. What happens then is that both partners end up resenting their loss of freedom. The truth is, the more intimate you are, the more freedom you both have to be yourselves. To get in touch with your ability to surrender to your partner, do the following written process:

1. My fears of totally surrendering to a man (woman) in an intimate sexual relationship are ________.
2. My fears of totally surrendering to being myself in the presence of a man (woman) are ________.
3. My fears of completely revealing myself to my intimate partner are ________.

You can write affirmations for any negative response you get. It would also be great to get rebirthed on the issues of intimacy, safety, trust and surrender.

Recently I did a One Day LRT with Philip and Mikela Tarlow, in Florida. We did a section on "doors to intimacy". I want to acknowledge their contribution to this material, and share it with you.

The first doorway to intimacy is verbal communication of the truth. Tell the truth faster, but don't process your partner, or tell them what is wrong with them, unless they ask for your support in that way. Take 100% responsibility for your relationship, especially if it isn't the way you want it to be.

The second doorway is going for the highest thought in your relationship. The highest thought is the least limiting, the most loving, and feels the best in your body. When deciding something that effects both you and your partner, you should both agree on the decision, or if you can't, keep thinking up new solutions until one of you has the highest thought that you both can agree on.

The third doorway is to share experiences from a common ground. See the similarities between you and your partner, instead of the differences. When sharing feelings, listen to your partner without judgement. Listening is the better part of communication. Often people just need someone to hear them, and not give any advice on how to handle the situation. If you just listen, you give your partner the opportunity to come up with their own solution. This empowers them.

The fourth doorway is to release your guilt, and experience your divine innocence. Play together, and have fun as you did as children. Reclaim your childlike innocence.

The fifth doorway to intimacy is compassion: understanding what your partner feels. Release your addiction to being right. Let go of your end of the rope. This is the easiest way to end fighting and conflict in a relationship. The more you fight about who is right, the less intimate you are.

The sixth doorway is to acknowledge your partner nightly. Acknowledgement is a turn-on to you and your partner. Get turned-on to your own magnificence, and the magnificence of your partner.

The seventh doorway is sharing your passion physically, emotionally, mentally and spiritually. Share your passion and enthusiasm for what you love to do, and for life, with your partner.

The eighth doorway is sharing sensuality. Take baths together; touch each other more; massage each other. Colognes and perfumes are very sensuous. Feel good and smell good. Get your skin to feel soft and silky. Arouse all your senses with each other.

The ninth doorway is both people having high self-esteem. That means that each person lives their Eternal Law, and loves themself in the presence of the other. Become the person you are looking for. Become two full cups, rather than two half-filled cups. The latter creates a relationship based on need: since you don't feel whole and complete, you need your partner to fulfill you. Being a full cup allows you to feel great, and have fun either alone, or together with your partner.

Someone who has mastered intimacy has the following characteristics:

1. Loves themselves unconditionally. That includes loving their body, and loving theirself as a male or a female.

2. Has ever increasing self-esteem, and feels they deserve infinite love. You will only let in as much love as you are willing to receive.

3. Is able to experience increasing amounts of pleasure and aliveness in their body. They are able to go past comfort zones: they notice when and where they want to cut off feelings. They communicate their fear of going beyond their comfort zone to their partner. This communication keeps the passion going, and allows them both to move past their fears of really being intimate.

4. Is willing to continually release separation issues, and dissolve boundaries between themselves and their partner. Becomes more and more at one with partner by being more and more compassionate, and letting go of all judgements.

5. Continually goes past their fear of loss. Passion, excitement, and safety take them beyond their fear of loss.

6. Is willing to see their partner as their guru or teacher. Is able to see the other person as part of their own mind reflection as it is. Is able to be responsible for changing what they don't like in that reflection. They know they are constantly attracting, projecting, and manifesting their relationships to be just as they believe they will be, based on their past decisions. They also know they can change their present reality by becoming conscious of their negative decisions, and changing them. They can do this by replacing the negative decisions with positive decisions, through the use of affirmations.
7. Is willing to continually be in present time, thus dissolving the past and not worrying about the future. This person has forgiven and released parents and siblings for past upsets, and is able to stay in present time with their parents and siblings.
8. Is willing to experience the totality of who they are; is living in their Eternal Law and is being their Divine self. They are living up to their full creative potential. Have released victim consciousness.

The affirmation for this chapter is "I am a beautiful, sexual, lovable man (woman), and I deserve to be loved to my core."

Sex and Communication

Sex is just another form of communicating with your partner. If you have great communication, the result is always great sex.

Having great communication with your partner means telling the truth faster. It means telling your partner everything: letting him or her know everything you need to clear in order to feel safe, supported, and thus able to surrender sexually.

Clearing with your partner does not mean blaming them or processing them about what is wrong with them. When you clear with someone, you use "I" sentences—"I feel this way," "I want to get closer to you, but what stands in the way is my fear of intimacy", etc. Taking 100% responsibility for what is going on in your relationship is what leads to clear communication.

There are several fun, easy games you can use to improve your communication with your partner. The Wet Truth Process, created by Bob and Mallie Mandel, is an excellent way to clear withholds. You and your partner sit in a hot bath facing each other. You each express how you feel, and how you are withholding love and energy from each other. You use "I" statements—"I feel like I can't get close to you," "I feel like I am pushed away," "I feel like my father pushed me away, and now you push me away," etc.. You stay in the tub until both of you have expressed everything that is between you, and you are feeling close and intimate again. Since you are extremely close and intimate in the hot water, this process works quickly and effectively. At the end of the bath, let the water and the withholds go down the drain.

Poopy Time, created by Peter and Meg Kane, allows you to get back into present time with your partner. If one person had a hard day and needs support, this is an excellent process to do. You give your partner ten minutes Poopy Time, when they can complain, bitch and moan. All the other person says is "Thank you", without making their partner wrong, or taking anything personally. This ten minutes allows you to support your partner, or be supported, while getting back into present time. Sometimes, all we need is for someone to listen to us, without giving us any of their great ideas.

If you have a right/wrong issue with your partner, which creates a lot of bickering and fighting, The Right Game is a good way to heal it. Often, people who have the Personal Lie that they are wrong, will have a big investment in being RIGHT. Peter Kane once told me, "If you are not willing to be wrong, you will never release your Personal Lie". We all have to be willing to be wrong about the negative decisions we made about ourselves. Hearing this helped me stop fighting, arguing, and wanting to prove I was always right. The Right Game helps to release the charge in letting your partner be right. This doesn't mean you have to feel like you are wrong.

The way the game is played is that one partner is allowed to be right about everything for one whole day. If they say the sky is green, you say, "That's right". You will notice that it gets easier and easier for you to let them be right without feeling wrong yourself. You will no longer have an investment in making your partner wrong, or in being right. Switch roles on another day: let the other partner be right all day long.

It's good to get into the practice of communicating, or doing a process with your partner, each night before going to sleep. Never go to sleep upset with each other. When you go to sleep upset, often you'll have bad dreams. And the longer you wait to clear issues, the harder it is to release them. When you stay in present time with your partner, the communication is always better, and so is the sex. Here are several processes you can do before going to sleep.

Forgiveness is the Master Erase and is very healing. You can say to your partner, "Something I forgive myself for in your presence is __________," and "Something I forgive you for is __________". Say these statements back and forth to each other until you both feel complete.

Acknowledgement always works, and is a great turn-on. "Something I love about you is __________". Each partner does five minutes of acknowledgement to their partner. You both will feel so great, you won't be able to wait to make love.

Below is another process that is good to do together in order to stay in present time, and keep communicating openly. Each person shares one round of all three statements, switching back and forth until you both feel complete.

Something I pray for is ________.

Something I forgive myself for is ________.

Something I am grateful for is ________.

Sondra Ray likes to include reading a *Course In Miracles* section together daily. This keeps you loving, close and connected. It is hard to feel separate from each other if you are healing your own personal separation issue with God.

I also like to remind myself often that Jeff is my guru, and acknowledge him frequently for all that he helps me to heal. Because love brings up everything unlike itself, for the purpose of healing and release, the more loved we are by our mate, the more negative, supressed decisions we will bring up for healing, with the help of our partner. Sometimes we can feel angry at our partners because we feel it is they who are making us feel uncomfortable. But if we acknowledge them for loving us and healing us, we can release the "unlike-it stuff" a lot easier and faster. We should also acknowledge them for allowing us to feel safe enough to allow so much to come up for healing.

Once you get your verbal communication handled with your partner, it is easier to ask for what you want sexually. Many people don't know what they want sexually. When I discovered that I really did not know what I wanted sexually, I started masturbating, and by trial and error with my partners, I finally discovered what it was that I wanted. Once I got in touch with what I wanted and what turned me on, I had to feel safe enough to ask my partner. I used to feel that it wasn't OK to ask for what I wanted. I know now that I felt I didn't deserve to get what I wanted, because I wasn't what may parents wanted. I now know that I am what I want, and since I know I am wanted by my partner, it is safe and easy to ask for, and get, what I want.

It is OK to ask to be touched softer, harder, slower, faster. It's OK to ask to be touched, stroked, or kissed in places that you feel sensitive. Only you know your own body.

I used to think that if my partner didn't know how to turn me on, then there must be something wrong with him and me. If you know what turns you on, let your partner know. Why keep it a secret, when you can get pleasure faster? Your partner could discover your sensitive spots on his or her own, but it could take a long time, and by then you could both be frustrated.

After you discover what turns you on, write it down. Also write down a fantasy you would like to act out. You can also include a position you have never tried and would like to try. Then write down all your fears of communicating all this to your partner. Tell your partner all your fears of communicating what you want sexually. Once you have told him/her your fears of communicating, actually telling him/her what you want will be easy. You will be amazed at how easy it is, and how wonderful and easy sex will become in your life.

Tell the truth faster in sex. Don't pretend you are having pleasure or orgasms if you are not. If you lie to your partner, you are really lying to yourself. You are blocking pleasure and orgasms. Since I felt like a disappointment as a woman, I would judge myself, thinking I was taking too much time. When I felt my partner was ready for an orgasm, I would pretend to have one. I was lying to my partner, and I was ripping myself off from having pleasure.

It's OK and great to talk during sex. Often people feel they have to be quiet during sex. It's much more of a turn on if you let your partner know how you are doing. You can communicate a lot through sounds. AHHHHH! UMMMMMM! OHHHHHHH! These are all good communicators of sexual bliss. Also, you can communicate by saying, "That feels good," "That feels great," "Touch me more," "Kiss me more", etc.. Lots of people get turned on by "talking dirty", like saying, "Fuck me," or "Fuck me harder". Experiment and see what turns you and your partner on the most.

Communication is an important key to a great sex life: master it and you will master your own sexuality.

Affirmations

1. It is easy to tell my partner the truth.
2. It's safe to communicate everything to my partner.
3. It's safe to communicate what I want sexually to my partner.
4. The more I communicate what I want sexually, the more I get it.
5. It's sexy to communicate during sex.
6. It's a turn on talk during sex.
7. Acknowledgement is a turn on during sex.
8. I know what I want sexually, and it's safe and easy to communicate it to my partner.

9. My partner wants to give me what I want sexually.
10. I deserve what I want sexually.
11. Communication is safe, easy and sexy.
12. I know how to communicate.
13. I get what I want when I communicate.
14. I love for my partner to tell me what he/she wants.

Love Your Sexual Body

The more you love and pleasure your body, the more pleasure you will have in sex. The more you tell your body you love it, the more your body will respond, act, and look the way you want it to. One way to achieve a beautiful, sexy body is to take five minutes a day in front of the mirror acknowledging it.

Stand nude in front of the mirror and say the following, "I love my hair, I love my face, I love my mouth, I love my neck, I love my shoulders, I love my feet." Proceed through your whole body, letting each part of your body know you love and appreciate it. Acknowledge your love for the parts that you don't like as they are, and then give them instructions to change. For example, "I love my tummy, and I would like you to be flatter." "I love my waist, and I would like you to be 25 inches around". Start to remold your body. The more your body pleases you, the more it will please your partner. The more it pleases your partner, the more it will please you and turn you on.

Over the past few years, I started to gain quite a bit of weight on my stomach, waist, hips, and thighs. I gained about 24 pounds, and 40 inches, overall. The reasons I carried the weight on these parts of my body was because I felt guilty about being a girl instead of a boy, and so I could be wrong as a woman. Sometimes I would get heavier if I were travelling a lot, and away from Jeff. I felt that if I was fat, men wouldn't want me or flirt with me. Men still flirted with me. The truth was that I needed to learn to be able to be thin and attractive, and at the same time to be able to say "no" to men that I didn't want to be attracted to me.

Many people use weight to protect themselves from intimacy. It is safe to be intimate, and it is safe and easy to say "no" to the people you don't want to be intimate with.

Also, I got fat after having an affair, because I felt guilty. Guilt demands punishment, so I got fat to punish myself. I believe that I get fat to hide my beauty and sexuality, just like my mother did, since my mother was my sexual role model. When she was heavy, it was always on her stomach and waist.

The more you affirm how beautiful your body is, the more sexy you will be and feel. You will also be able to experience more pleasure in your body. Often we use our body as an excuse for not being intimate and sexy. "If only I were thin, I would have a great sex life." If you get thin, then you can no longer use this as an excuse not to have pleasurable, exciting sex.

Your body is like your home and car; it represents who you are. Your body should represent your highest thought about yourself: "I am a beautiful, lovable man (woman), and I deserve to be loved," not your lowest thought about yourself: "I am not good enough" or "I am not wanted". It takes high self-esteem to have a beautiful body and keep it. You have to be willing to love yourself as much as everyone else does. Often, people lose a lot of weight, and then gain it all back. This is because they do not love themselves enough to be beautiful and thin.

Often we think that food makes us fat. The reality is that our thoughts make us fat. Our thoughts about our body, ourselves, intimacy, sex, and food make us fat. Read *The Only Diet There Is* by Sondra Ray. This book helps you to clear your thoughts about food and yourself, so you can lose weight. It helps you to lighten up your thoughts, which helps to lighten up your body.

Recently I lost 18 pounds and 40 inches. I lost the weight because I was ready to integrate the belief that I was an innocent, sexual, pleasurable, and attractive woman, who was wanted and appreciated by men. It is important to change your thoughts about yourself, food, sex, intimacy, and your body, so that you can accept your new body image as you achieve it.

It is also important to really understand that when you are thin and sexy, you can say "no" to people you do not want to be intimate with. You can say "no" to people without losing their love. It is easier to say "no" then it is to lose weight. I have noticed that it usually takes me three or four months to lose the weight I gained because I thought I didn't know how to say "no".

Besides changing my thoughts about being a sexy, beautiful, thin woman, and my thoughts about food, I acted on three techniques for weight loss that gave me the results I wanted. Changing our thoughts is the feminine, intuitive aspect of creating change. I also used my masculine side to create my desired results: I took action.

I did European body wrapping. This was the incentive I needed to get started and discipline myself. The first time, I lost eight inches over my whole body. This method is so simple that people won't try it, because they think it is too easy. People who are in a struggle pattern will not try anything that they think is easy. They think they have to work hard to lose weight.

In this method, they wrap you in hot, white bandages which are soaked in minerals which break down the cellulite and fatty tissue. They guarantee that you will lose 6 to 2 inches from the first wrap, or you get your money back. The loss is permanent, as long as you maintain your weight or lose weight. I lost thirty inches, doing this twice a week for about seven weeks.

You drink eight to ten glasses of water a day. This helps to break down the fat and detoxify your body. When the bandages are on you, you have a plastic suit on to keep the heat in, and you relax for an hour. While I was relaxing, I would listen to Sondra Ray's tape "Your Ideal Loving Relationship With Your Body and Weight." This way I was changing my thoughts and my body at the same time.

Also, I love to work out at the gym. I would go and ride the lifecycle bicycle for aerobic exercise for twelve minutes to one hour, depending on how busy I was. During the time I was riding the bike, I listened to Sondra's weight tape and other enlightened tapes, and read either enlightened books or romances that would turn me on. I made getting my body back into shape fun, and utilized the time to change my thoughts with enlightened, metaphysical books. I did a weight program too, to firm my legs, stomach, waist, back, arms, and chest. When I had extra time, I loved to swim 25 laps in the pool, and take a jacuzzi, steam or sauna.

After I left the gym I felt really alive, sexual, and energized. Before I lost weight, I could hardly walk up and down the three flights of stairs in my house without having trouble breathing. This was when I knew I had to do something, because I didn't feel alive and energized like I normally did. I was too busy to notice that I had gotten fat and out of shape.

I also joined Weight Watchers, which was great for me. I lost nine pounds in five weeks. I noticed that I usually gained weight when I went out of town and travelled, teaching the LRT. Weight Watchers gave me balanced meals which I could eat and still lose weight. I found I could eat more than I usually ate if I was on a diet, and still lose weight. They give you three balanced meals a day.

My tendency before doing Weight Watchers would be to starve myself all day, and then eat one large meal in the evening, and usually stuff myself. Weight Watchers gives you new eating habits that are very satisfying. I didn't feel like I was denying myself anything. You can eat lots of popcorn, and they have great deserts, if you have a sweet tooth. The weekly meetings are very helpful in keeping you on the program.

I am sharing what worked for me to help you find out what works for you. Self-discipline is very important in getting to your weight loss goal. Having a support system like Weight Watchers helps in staying on your own personal program that works for you. Another reason I tried everything available was so that I could share with people what had worked for me.

I have noticed that since my body is slimmer, I enjoy being touched more. Jeff loves touching me more, and my body responds better than ever.

How much you love your body is directly proportional to how much you will let your intimate partner love your body. Your body is your temple, and your vehicle for sexual pleasure. It is important to love and respect your body, and treat it like the temple it is. If you don't love and respect your body, it will break down and not function up to its full capacity, just as a car breaks down when it doesn't get oil, gas and water.

To have your body give you all the pleasure you deserve, you have to feed it well-balanced, nutritional foods from the six basic food groups: dairy, protein, grains, fats, vegetables, and fruits. You also have to give it the right instructions mentally in order to have it be its perfect weight and body proportions. It's important to get regular exercise too. Eight to ten glasses of water a day helps to flush toxins out of your body, and to reach and maintain your ideal weight.

The most important thing is to eat when you are hungry. Eat to pleasure yourself if you want, but be aware that you are using food to replace love. Find the love instead of eating the food. Often, our parents gave us food instead of love, so later on in life we use food as a substitute for love. The more you become aware of doing this, the easier it is to stop overeating, and ask for what you want from your lover and friends.

Ways to Pleasure and Love Your Body

Massage

Chiropractic treatment

Deep tissue massage, Rolfing, Heller Work, Body Harmony

Rebirthing

Hot bubble bath and hot mineral bath

Herbal bath

Mineral herbal body wrap

Aerobic workout

Nautilis equipment workout

Facial

Hiking, running, tennis, racketball

Masturbation

Dancing

Sex

Jacuzzi and hot tub

Written Process

My thoughts about my body are ________.

When I weigh ________, I will ________.

Whatever you said you will do, do it now; don't wait. You will get to your ideal weight faster if you pleasure yourself on the way, and make it a fun and exciting adventure. Living your life as you are changing your body, is better than waiting to live until you have created your ideal body. You might have to wait a long time to be in the present moment, which is the best time there is.

Affirmations for a Beautiful, Sexy Body

1. I love, accept and approve of my body exactly the way it is.
2. I have the perfect body.
3. My body is innocent.
4. I am innocent for having a sexual body.
5. My body listens to my instructions.
6. I now weigh my ideal perfect weight of ________.
7. My body is pleasing to myself.
8. My body is pleasing to myself in the presence of others.
9. It's safe for me to have a thin, sexy body.
10. My body gives me pleasure.
11. The thinner and more beautiful my body is, the easier it is to say "no" to what I don't want sexually.

Creating Exciting Sexual Adventures

Creating exciting, sexual adventures can be a lot of fun and a real turn on. It is important to be in touch with what you really want sexually, in order to receive it. Sexual fantasies are healthy, unless they get in the way of achieving pleasure with your partner. If your fantasy becomes something that takes you away from bliss and pleasure with your partner, you may want to let it go, and find an exciting sexual adventure that you could create together.

Writing out your ideal sexual experience or fantasy can be quite thrilling, and help bring new magic into your relationship. Once you have written down your ideal sexual experience or fantasy, read it to your partner, and then have fun acting it out. If you have fears of communicating it to your partner, tell him or her your fears, and then move through them.

In this chapter there are several descriptions of ideal sexual experiences and fantasies. There are included to give you new ideas, and get you excited about creating your own ideal experiences and fantasies.

There are also some suggestions of unusual locations for having sex, to spice up your relationship. I think all of us like to have sex in unusual places, with the little bit of danger of being found or caught. Sex can become boring and unexciting if we always make love with the same person, in the same way, in the same place. Instead of giving up your partner to get more variety, think of giving up the same old positions, places, and routines. Have "mini-moons", or little one-night, two-day vacations. Go to fun places such as the beach, mountains, desert, hot springs, lakes, rivers or any little, new hideaway you find. This will keep the romance alive in your relationship.

Unusual Locations for Sex

On a houseboat.

On a sailboat.

On a motor boat cruiser.

On the deck of a cruise boat.

Mile high club—in the friendly skies.

On a football field.

On a baseball field.

On a golf course.

On a tennis court.

On a ski slope.

In the Senate Chambers.

In the middle of an icy cliff in February, hanging off a ledge.

On a desert island.

In a carwash.

In a glass elevator.

In a plush restaurant.

On a horse.

On a motorcycle, driving in Alligator Alley.

In a deserted car.

In a subway.

In a cave.

In an ocean.

On a raft, going down a river.

In an amusement park.

In a jacuzzi.

On the beach.

On top of a mountain.

In the desert.

On a sand dune.

In the back seat of your parents' car, when your parents are in it.

In a swimming pool.

Under a waterfall.

On your front lawn.

Sexual Fantasy with a Policeman

I am driving my red convertible down the Pacific Coast Highway, just as sunset is hitting the Malibu beaches. I have the top down, and it is still warm, with the wind swirling my hair around my face. I have on a light sundress, with no underwear underneath. George Michael's tape "Faith, I Want Your Sex" is blasting on my stereo. I start to feel really turned on. I reach underneath my dress and start playing with myself. I begin to get very, very hot and wet. I start touching myself faster and faster, when all of a sudden I come back to present time, and look at my speedometer. I am going eighty-five miles an hour. Before I can slow down, a cop on a motorcycle pulls up behind me, flashing his lights. Still feeling hot and turned on, I pull over.

I get out of the car, and standing beside me is one of the best-looking men I have ever seen. He is over six feet tall; a blue-eyed blond with a wonderful body. I smile at him innocently. He says very sharply, "Young lady, do you realize how fast you were going?" I look up at him with a smile and say, "I was having so much fun that I didn't really notice how fast I was going 'til right when you stopped me." He asks me, "What were you having fun with?" I tell him I was enjoying the sunset, George Michael, and pleasuring my body. He sees my flushed cheeks, and knows exactly what I mean.

He takes my arm, walks me over to the beach, and passionately starts kissing me. It feels so good I can't say "no". I am still so turned on from earlier. He starts kissing me all over, licking me with his tongue. He kisses and licks my breasts as he lifts my dress and touches my clitoris. I feel his warm body against me, his gun and his penis both very hard against my body. He pulls me down on the sand, and quickly pulls his pants down and is inside me before I know what's happening. I am already so turned on that I have one orgasm after another before he finally is satisfied. We get up and he says, "Lady, you had better slow down next time. You were so nice that I won't give you a ticket this time, but this is a warning." He jumps back on his motorcycle and speeds off.

Sexual Fantasy of Giving My Partner Total Pleasure

I am at home with my boyfriend, and it is raining as usual. We both feel bored, and want to do something different. I have always wanted to tie him to the bedposts and make love to him. Today, he is as bored as I am, and readily agrees. We go down to my daughter's bedroom—she is spending the night at a girlfriend's. She has a four-poster bed. I tie his legs and arms spread-eagle to the bed. He is already undressed. I have on a soft, silk teddy.

The first thing I do is take our feather duster and tickle him lightly all over his body, to get him aroused. Then I take some warm oil and give him a foot, leg, chest, and neck rub. Then I start licking his toes, taking each one in my mouth and sucking it. This always turns him on. By now he is squirming, and almost can't stand receiving so much pleasure. Then I take some

Cool Whip, and spread it all over his penis and genital area. I slowly and lusciously lick it off. He can hardly hold himself back any longer; he really wants to come, or please me. I just tell him to keep breathing. He takes some deep breaths, and then he is ready to receive more pleasure.

I start rubbing my breasts all over his body, starting with his penis and slowly working my way upward. I finally get my breasts up to his mouth and he slowly starts licking them exactly the way I love them licked. I am already turned on by his moans and groans, and his obvious pleasure in what I have been doing to him for the last hour. He can hardly contain himself any longer.

Again he starts to breathe, and is able to sustain his pleasure, and even have it get more intense. I get on top of him. I have taken off my teddy, and I sit on top of his penis and slowly ride him. We are looking into each other's eyes, and we see the depths of who we each are. We begin to merge into each other, no longer feeling any separation between us. We are one, and feel one sensation: the pleasure that is sweeping over both of us simultaneously. We both experience pink, purple, and white lights as we cry out in ecstasy.

Sexual Fantasy with Buddha

I am lying naked on my bed under an open window. I am feeling turned-on by the cool breeze flowing over me. Trying to be serious, I focus on my meditation, visualizing my ideal career.

I can't concentrate. The wind is sensually tracing every inch of my body from my head to my feet. Now someone is licking my toes. This can't be. I am all alone. I open my eyes, and am startled by the aura of a man. I think "Wow, I've got to stop meditating so often. It's making me hallucinate." The figure begins to fill in, and it looks like BUDDHA! Jumping up, I cry "Buddha, what are you doing here?" But Buddha prevents me from getting up by placing his body on top of mine. I try to resist, but his body touching mine soothes my muscles so much that I have no choice except to relax under him.

All these thoughts come to my mind, "Oh my God, this is Buddha. I can't do this. I should be on my knees, not on my back." Buddha hears my thoughts, and whispers to me as he lusciously licks my ear, "I've been listening to your fantasies for a long time. I know exactly what you want, how you like it, and for how long you like it." I begin to speak, but he interrupts me and says, "You don't need to say or do anything. You created me, and I hear every thought in your head. My desire is to fulfill you."

A trusting, loving sensation envelopes my body. I lie back in the comfort of knowing that every delicious thought I have ever fantasized is about to come true.

Sexual Fantasy at the Beach

In the calm waters, we are swimming nude and playing with dolphins. It's Kauai, or somewhere remote in the Caribbean. Our dogs are lying on the beach, watching and waiting for us. It's mid-afternoon. We take a break in the shade of some palm trees. We start talking softly, giggling and gently caressing each other. I draw little lines with my fingers over his stomach, chest and legs. He moves his fingers down my neck, shoulders and back. In between conversations, we kiss, alternating long probing tongues with little flickering movements. One of us makes a silly noise, and we collapse with laughter and begin tickling each other. Then we get hot again, and start erotically playing up and down each other's inner thighs with fingers and tongues. We take turns with our mouths on each other's genitals, gently touching with our fingers as we do. There are funny noises and laughter. I am laughing as I come. He gets close several times, but wants to wait. We take a break, and give each other back and neck massages.

We are talking about God, and how we want to feel God with us and through us while we make love. This gets us excited again. He comes inside me, starting on top of me and thrusting very slowly. My insides are melting into his, and we are making little noises at each other, in some pre-verbal conversation. It is as if we are both meditating, almost still. We start breathing together, connectedly. We roll over so I am on top. I am making small movements and contractions, just enough to keep him excited. His head is back, his eyes are closed, and he is moaning and crying. I am very hot, but I keep breathing, and I keep the movements slow.

By now, I can see the last of the sunset over the water. It is an incredible band of color, and I cry with joy. The dogs lie nearby, watching silently, cheering us on. He decides he wants to come. He wants me from behind. I'm ready. As he enters me, I start these rapid spasms. I feel like they will never stop. I can no longer tell what is me and what is him. We are all one, fluid whole. We are making all kinds of noises. Thank God the beach is deserted!

Then things slow down. He rests his head on my back, holding my breasts for support. Soon my elbows give out and we both fall into the sand. That starts us giggling, so we re-arrange ourselves and cuddle, gently caressing random places on each other and taking quietly. Eventually we decide it's either sleep or swim, so we race into the water, shouting, splashing, dunking and laughing. By now it is totally dark, the stars and moon are up, and we can hear the night birds singing. We float for a while, holding hands. Then we go home for some food.

Sexual Fantasy on a Stallion

My favorite sexual fantasy is of making love on the back of a powerful stallion. My partner and I begin by galloping across the desert. We fly along, getting more and more excited, feeling one with the wind. I am sitting in front of him, and he begins nibbling on my neck. As he gently caresses my breasts, my excitement mounts. I urge him to take me now! I lean over the neck of the stallion while he eases my dress up over my waist. He enters me from behind, and I lean back. The movement of the horse enhances our rhythm. We come together as the stallion pounds across the sandy floor.

Sexual Fantasy at a Sex Research Lab

I sometimes visualize this fantasy when I masturbate. I am lying on a massage table in a beautiful room in a sex research lab. I have been hired to participate in some research studies on arousal and orgasms. There is a large two-way mirror on the wall. There are several machines around the table, and one hanging from the ceiling. There is a man behind the mirror who instructs me as to what to do. He can see me, but I am blindfolded.

Some gentle music comes on, and I hear the click of the machines as they turn on. I resist with the thought that I won't be turned on by any machine. Soft rubbery hands caress my breasts, and then a medium-sized rubber penis starts rubbing up and down on my vagina. I squirm around and resist some more. The gentle voice from behind me says, "Relax, let's just give it a few minutes to see what happens." I squirm and resist some more. I tell him "This is not working." In my mind I know that it could, but I really want him. I complain that the machine is not placed properly, and I ask him to come and adjust it. I know that he is not allowed, but I want to tease and tempt him. A few more minutes go by, and I tell him again that I need help. He says he could lose his job if he enters the room. I promise I won't tell.

I hear the door open and he enters. Excited now, I hear him come closer. I feel his leg brush against me as he fiddles with the machine. I start telling him how much it would help me get more in the mood, if I could just touch him. He resists verbally, but he doesn't move away. I reach out, still blindfolded, and gently stroke his penis. Slowly, I unzip his pants. I loosen them down gently, and pull him toward me. He still resists. His fear of getting caught is strong. As I put his penis gently in my mouth, he surrenders. He's mine now. His passion is overwhelming his body. We proceed to fondle and caress each other from head to toe. I make love, I have an orgasm, I fall asleep.

Belly Dancing Fantasy

I have always had a fascination with the idea of being in a harem. I decided to take a belly dancing class, so I could sexually arouse my boyfriend and myself. After six weeks of practising my erotic, exotic movements, I finally got the pelvic and hip motions good enough to try out my enticement on my boyfriend. I had kept what I was doing every Tuesday night for six weeks a secret from him, so I could surprise him. Finally, the right night came. I set the mood by putting candles all over the bedroom, and burning incense. I put on the music, and put on my sexy, belly dancing outfit. I noticed that all the practicing had really slimmed down my waist and hips.

I started gyrating my hips and pelvis as I clicked my finger symbols. I immediately got my boyfriend's attention away from the sports page he was reading. He watched my hips and pelvis as I started shaking them all over the place. I had all the right moves for my hips, pelvis, breasts, hands and legs. He started breathing harder as he watched me dance before him. I went closer, and ran my silky outfit gently over his body, touching him just enough to create goosebumps. He started to grab me, but I wasn't through yet. I knew the next part was even more sensuous.

I got down on the floor and started slithering back and forth, kissing and licking his toes. I continued shaking my breasts in front of him. He could stand it no longer, and reached to squeeze and fondle my breast, which just made my movement more frantic and intense. The more turned on he became, the more animal-like my movements became. I no longer was in control of my body. I was shaking in an involuntary way, making groaning and moaning sounds.

My partner could not stand the excitement he felt any longer. His penis was bulging and pulsating with passion and excitement. I took him totally by surprise with my new-found talent. He grabbed my leg and pulled me to the floor. He rolled me over so that I could get on my hands and knees in front of him. He started kissing my neck, and rubbing his hard penis up and down my back. As he licked my ear and told me he loved me, he started stroking my breasts until I had my first orgasm. Then he entered me from behind. The feelings were the most intense I had ever had. I felt as though I would burst open. I felt both pleasure and pain. My body wanted more. We were both dripping with sweat.

As I had another orgasm, he turned me over on my back so that he could look into my eyes. He came inside me, and looked adoringly at me for providing such an erotic adventure. Just looking into my eyes, and seeing how excited I was, pushed him over into his own bliss, and we came together with such intensity that it was hard to breathe. Our bodies melted together, and we merged into each other. We felt that feeling we love so much of being truly connected on a soul level. I smiled, acknowledging myself for keeping my little secret, and for how wonderfully it had all turned out.

The Effects of Feminism on Sexuality

The feminist movement has effected the sex lives of both men and women. "Women wanting equal rights" means more than just equal rights in the work force. Women also want equal rights sexually.

In the traditional family of the past, sex was for the pleasure of the man. Often, sex was a duty for the woman, performed in exchange for being taken care of financially by the man. Women birthed and raised the children, took care of the home, cooked and cleaned. The men worked and brought in the paycheck. If women were pleasured and satisfied sexually that was okay, but not necessary.

As women have begun to enter the work force and make their own livings, they have also been more demanding in the bedroom. Women want pleasure, orgasms, bliss and sexual excitement too.

Men and women often want different things sexually. Since the feminist movement, men are learning more and more that women want to be sexually satisfied. Women are more outspoken now about what they want sexually; they see sexual pleasure as their right. Equal rights in the bedroom is an important issue.

Women often like more cuddling, affection, romance and foreplay than men. Men often like quick sex, and this doesn't always please women. Men are finding that as they slow down and please women, they often discover that they like more affection, cuddling, romance and foreplay too. Men are learning from women that slower sex can be better, because it builds up the energy and excitement.

I was raised in a traditional family. I thought my role was to please a man, and consequently he would take care of me financially and emotionally. I didn't have orgasms. I was so busy pleasing my partners, I didn't please myself. I would pretend I had orgasms, and that I was excited, so my partner would be pleased with me, and not disappointed in me as a woman. I didn't feel that I deserved the time it took to please me. Just as I had not taken the time to know what pleasured me, I didn't give myself the time I needed to enjoy sex, and be orgasmic.

The fact that women are demanding sexual pleasure from men can seem scary to men at first, because they are used to being pleased instead of pleasing. Once men learn how to pleasure their partners, however, they see that sex is even more satisfying and pleasurable than in the past. When both partners are pleased, sex is much more satisfying.

When both partners have high self-esteem, it is easy for them to ask for, and receive, what they want sexually. The feminist movement has moved men and women more into balance. Both women and men are learning how to give and receive. Giving and receiving, the male and female, the Yin and Yang, is what brings about orgasmic, mutually satisfying sex.

Balancing Male and Female Energy

One of the keys to having a great sexual relationship is to balance your male and female energy. People usually project more of one energy than the other.

Since my parents wanted a boy, I learned a lot about being a boy to please them. I cultivated my male energy more than my female energy, because that is what I thought my parents wanted.

Male energy is assertive, goes for what it wants, comes from the intellect, is precise, planned, exacting, giving, providing, aggressive, and forceful. Males are not afraid to ask for what they want, and make things happen. The male part of us is the part that gets things done. The male part of us is the initiator, or giver, in sex.

I was great at initiating and giving in sex, but terrible about receiving. As I rebirthed and did the LRT, I began to love and accept myself as a woman. I started pampering myself; giving myself facials, massages, manicures, working out, and dressing more sexily and feminine. As I worked on a more feminine appearance, my female energy stated to come more into balance. I became softer, and got what I wanted a lot more easily.

Female energy is creative, soft, intuitive, shares feelings easily, comes from the heart, receives well, nurtures, and knows the right things to do instinctively. The female part of us is the creative, intuitive part, which needs the male energy to really make things happen. The female part of us creates the decisions, and the male part of us takes action to make the ideas a reality.

It is important for each of us to balance and harmonize our own female and male energies. Otherwise, we must depend on another person to make us feel whole and complete. As our energy comes into balance, sex becomes more exciting and less routine. At any given moment, either person can be the initiating giver, or the creative receiver.

When our energy is balanced. We can let go of the resentment of feeling we need another person to complete us, or make us whole. We are complete, whether we are apart or together. Instead of two half cups coming together, we are two full cups. Being two full cups gives us more excitement, energy and love.

Affirmations

1. My male and female energies are in balance.
2. I am a full cup.
3. It's safe to be a receiver and a giver.
4. It's safe to initiate sex.
5. Being balanced gives me freedom.

Rebirthing and Sex

Rebirthing makes sex so easy and enjoyable. Most people have a tendency to hold their breath when making love. When we hold our breath, we hold back pleasure and hold in pain. When you start breathing, you feel more energy, more aliveness, and of course the result is more pleasure.

Sex is rebirthing. If you start breathing a lot when you are excited, you will have a feeling of letting go, forgetting your boundaries, and you will allow yourself to be at one with your partner. You will move from past time or future time into the present moment, and into the immortal mind of feeling at-one with yourself, God, and your partner.

Rebirthers are initially surprised at this side benefit of rebirthing. Sex gets better and better. This makes perfect sense, since as I have said throughout this book, our birth and conception affects our sexuality. It is perfectly logical that the more we rebirth, and clear our birth trauma and our death urge, the safer and more exciting sex will become. As we release anesthesia, unconsciousness, pain, resentment, fear, guilt, anger and sadness from the cells of our body, our body wakes up and becomes more sensitive: more full of sexually alive and innocent energy.

Rebirthing is our tool in the LRT for releasing all the garbage we have accumulated throughout our lives. The breath allows us to take in more energy, aliveness and love, and breathe out the negativity, pain, anger, guilt, and sadness. It's a simple process, and it works to heal us in all areas. For me, sexuality was my biggest issue. Even without focusing on this issue—just by rebirthing and doing LRT trainings—I was able to experience things sexually that I had never been able to before. I have been rebirthing for nine years, and sex gets better and better. (See Appendix B for information on how to choose and find a rebirther in your area.)

Sex and Marriage

I knew that writing a chapter on sex and marriage was important. Doing this chapter myself seemed difficult. I have not been married for nine years, and sex in my marriage was very difficult. Consequently, this chapter has been one of the last to be completed.

I was trying to avoid this topic, and thought I had already completed the book. Recently, while I was in India, I asked Shastriji, a clairvoyant and saint who is the mouthpiece of Babaji, if this book would be a success. He told me the book would be a complete success, but I still had three chapters to write. He said I knew what these chapters were, and I had been avoiding writing them.

Earlier, I had asked Mallie and Bob Mandel to contribute a chapter on sex and marriage because I felt they were the experts on this topic within the LRT organization. Because of busy schedules, and my lack of certainty on including this chapter, they had not written their contribution until now.

Because I did not have Bob and Mallie's chapter, I decided to interview several couples within the LRT community, in order to shed some light on how to write this chapter. I interviewed these couples about their sex lives before and after marriage. We also discussed how their conceptions, womb periods, births and Personal Lies affected their sex lives.

Before I share these interviews, and Mallie and Bob's section with you, I would like to share briefly about my sex life within my marriage.

I was married for eight years. I had a good sex life with my husband before I was married to him. At least, my sex life seemed good to me at the time, for it was the best sex I had experienced up to then. I had had limited sexual experience.

My husband had been very sexual before he and I got together. He really wanted to please me sexually, and he knew how to do it. As I stated previously in this book, I went many years without orgasms. Before I met my husband, I had only had orgasms when I masturbated. I was able to have an orgasm with my husband when we had oral sex, but not in intercourse.

After we got married, our sex life diminished quite a bit and we were lucky if we made love once a month. Since he was extremely active sexually before me, he was frustrated with me sexually. I will admit now that I was very unconscious sexually, and not very sensitive. I really didn't care if we had sex or not; it was just not that important to me at the time. My husband had an affair which he did not tell me about for several years. Sex became the major problem in our marriage. We read books on how to improve our sex lives, we took tantric workshops, and we went to swing parties where we had other partners. We tried everything we could at the time to heal our sex life. Because we were unhappy about sex, we had other upsets resulting from the frustration and anger. These other upsets were about money, and about neither of us really receiving what we wanted from each other, and from the marriage.

Looking back on our sex life, after knowing everything I know now, I feel that I copied WHAT I THOUGHT MY PARENTS' SEX LIFE WAS, not the reality of their sex life. I thought my parents never had sex. I thought my parents were asexual, so this is what I created in my marriage. I created occasional sex, and sex to create two beautiful children. I also thought that my parents only had sex to create their three children. I created in my marriage the same thing that my parents communicated to me about their sex lives. I had no idea that sex was pleasurable, blissful, exciting or fun. My parents never communicated any of this to me about sex. Sex was a big secret that you found out about when you were married. During my marriage, I never seemed to discover the real truth about sex.

Eventually, our problems with sex created more affairs, a lot of anger, and the breakdown of our marriage. I understand now that because I had low self-esteem, I did not love and accept myself as a woman. I felt that I was a disappointment as a woman, especially sexually. I had a lot of sexual guilt. I did not know how to communicate about sex, or what I wanted sexually. If I somehow managed to communicate what I wanted sexually, I really didn't feel that I deserved it, because of my sexual guilt, and because of feeling not really wanted as a woman by my father and husband. It seemed like it was impossible to do anything other than fail in my marriage. Communication about your sex life in marriage is a key factor in having sex be comfortable, safe and exciting.

On other levels, my husband and I were very close. We spent almost twenty-four hours a day with each other. The more time we spent together, the less sexual we felt. Because we worked together, and spent every minute together, we found ourselves feeling less and less turned on to each other.

We set up the Suppressed Family Sexuality Pattern (incest pattern): the more we spent time together, the less attracted we felt, and the less we wanted to make love to each other. We became brothers, sisters, mothers and fathers to each other. When couples go through this, they usually make themselves wrong instead of recognizing the pattern.

What tends to happen in a marriage when sex breaks down, is each person blames the other for the problem. It is important for each partner to take responsibility for what is not working in the relationship sexually.

How is your conception affecting your sexuality? Were you wanted and planned as a man or woman? How does your birth affect your sexuality? How does your Personal Lie affect your sexuality? How does your parental conditioning affect your sexuality? How does your church conditioning affect your sexuality? How do your early nourishment patterns affect your sexuality?

If both people have the thought they can't have what they want sexually, these thoughts could come from not being breastfed and/or from being fed on a schedule. Each person in a relationship has to recognize the part they play in not having sex be the way they want it to be. GO FOR SOLUTION, AND LET GO OF THE BLAME. Couple consultations with another couple you trust, or with your rebirther, really help you to see the part each of you has in creating the sexual problem in your relationship. Often, we can only see our partner's issues, and not our own. This is a good time to have objective professional help to support you in healing your relationship together.

Acknowledgment and nightly clearing processes always work to re-establish the connection and closeness with your partner. Sometimes, we know what works to feel closer, but we resist because we have a lot of fear of intimacy and vulnerability. Often, people shut down sexually because they are afraid of allowing their partners to be so close and see them so deeply. FEAR FORWARD AND LET THE PAST GO, so that you can start over with your partner and create safe, passionate, cosmic, blissful, intimate and exciting sex.

Sex and Marriage Interview with Al and Nancy

The first thought that Al had about Nancy was that he was drawn to her loving energy. Nancy was afraid of her attraction to Al because she was still married at the time of their initial attraction. She was separated from her husband, but not legally divorced.

They had their first date in July, 1987. Al was told by a psychic to go to Mt. Shasta, because the woman of his dreams would be there. When Al saw Nancy, he knew that she was the one he wanted to meet. Nancy felt that she wasn't ready for a new relationship. She wanted to be friends and buddies. For the first week of the two-week course they were taking, they were just hugging each other like buddies. Nancy started to have fantasies about Al.

Al was trying to respect Nancy's feelings of not being ready for a relationship. At some point, they ended up nude, sunbathing and kissing each other. Once they were alone, and went with the energy they felt between them, they knew they wanted to be sexual with each other. They sneaked away to Nancy's tent, and kissed and touched each other. After they finally got together, they slept together for the next week.

Nancy went through her GUILT, and Al was IN LUST, and he thought he was IN LOVE. He was really enjoying Nancy and the connectedness they shared with each other.

When Nancy and Al had sex, Nancy was excited until penetration, then she got scared. She had made love for ten years to someone with a vasectomy. They weren't using birth control, so she had a fear of getting AIDS or getting pregnant. She had been celibate for two months before she met Al. She was scared and horny at the same time.

When they left each other after Mt. Shasta, Nancy visited Al and his whole family. She went home after that and sold her home, settled her divorce, and arranged to go back to live with Al.

Al told Nancy when they first met, "I want you to have my baby, and I want to marry you." Nancy felt that this was a clue from God that Al was the right man. This was the sign she was waiting for.

They had only known each other two weeks, but they had met each other two more times, once in Denver, and once in Knoxville. They had great sex on both these occasions.

They married on October 18, 1987, three months after they met. They conceived their baby October 25, 1987, one week after their wedding.

From July until October, making love together was connected and like making love to God. They saw Jesus, and the oneness of the universe. They would look into each other's eyes and see their souls when they reached orgasm. When they conceived their baby, they connected their eyes during intercourse, and they experienced the orgasm moving up and through them. They felt filled with light, and they felt the spirit of the baby filling both of them. After the baby was conceived, they had great sex while they were pregnant. Al would say, "The baby wants us to have sex."

In the third month of the pregnancy, Nancy started bleeding. She began having memories of her mother having a brother who died at birth. Her parents had made love the whole time this baby was in the womb. Nancy's mother later thought that making love had killed this baby. Nancy started dealing with these thoughts. She tried to believe that sex was healing and benefitting her baby. After the baby was born, they didn't have as good or as frequent sex. They worried about getting pregnant again before they were ready.

Nancy was a wanted and planned baby with a controlled conception. Her mother took her temperature so she would know when she was fertile. Nancy was seven and a half months in the womb. The waters broke, and sixteen hours later they decided to do a caesarean birth. She was separated from her mother for twenty-four hours. Nancy's mom wanted to nurse, but Nancy fell asleep at the breast and Nancy's mom's breasts became engorged. Then Nancy could not be nursed, and was put on a bottle. Nancy's Personal Lies are I AM A DISAPPOINTMENT and I CAN'T DO IT RIGHT.

Al's conception was wanted and planned. His birth was induced. He was late; he was in the womb ten months, and did not want to come out. They pulled him out with forceps. He feels that he has to hold back his aliveness, and he feels guilty for hurting his mother and other women.

In the beginning of their relationship, Al initiated sex. After they had been married awhile, their birth patterns came up. Now Nancy initiates sex, and Al wants to be induced.

Nancy resents always having to initiate sex, and is upset because she feels she is not getting what she wants. For her, not getting what she wants is related to not being nourished the way she wanted at her birth—with the breast. Now, she feels she is not nourished sexually. Initially, she got what she wanted sexually with Al, just like at birth she initially got the breast. Later, she had to settle for formula.

Al had sex outside his marriage in his last marriage. He has fears about performance, and not doing it right. His way of having sex has changed. Fantasy is what kept him excited in the past. He feels guilty about having to be induced sexually. He feels that he hurts Nancy in this way, like he hurt his mother at birth. Withholding coming out at his birth is what hurt his mother. Now, he withholds sex unless he is induced. When we relax in our marriages, we go on automatic and go right into our patterns.

Al wants GOD SEX now. He wants to love the one he is with—Nancy, be in the moment, and merge with her. When he doesn't feel these things sexually, he feels guilty. He feels that when they aren't having GOD SEX, they are acting out their Suppressed Incest Patterns. He feels that both of them are acting like their moms and dads when they don't feel connected, and forget who they are with. *Our partners are not our parents.* Al is starting to feel and see the real benefits of the deep connection and intimacy he has with Nancy.

For Al, sex has often been an afterthought, a result of guilt and pain. Often, guilt is so much on his mind he can't have sex, or when he does have sex, he is too guilty to allow the connection to happen. Al's goal for sex now is to stay connected and intimate with Nancy. This brings back the sexual desire.

There are some other conflicts in Nancy and Al's sex life. She likes morning sex, and he likes late night or noon sex. They also have the "baby incest pattern". The baby is always with them, and wants to be involved with whatever they are doing. The baby seems to know when they are feeling sexual, and either wakes up or is up already.

Nancy and Al have reported to me that since they talked about their sex life in this interview, they have had more sex, and feel more connected. Merely remembering their connection, passion and initial attraction, helped them to feel more connected and sexual with each other. What you focus on, expands. Focus on the passion, connectedness, and all the good you have enjoyed in your sex lives, so that you can create more of it.

Sex and Marriage Interview with Mark and Sue

Mark and Sue have been married eleven years. They dated for eleven months before they were married during which they traveled for three months in Europe.

They met at the art school that they were both attending. They knew each other for four months before they had sex and became intimate. They had a good friendship before they had sex. Sue knew the first week she met Mark that she loved him. It took Mark a longer time to realize he loved Sue.

When they were travelling together, Mark proposed marriage to Sue on the Irish Sea. Initially, Mark was more attracted to Sue as a friend, than sexually. The sexuality between them grew.

Before marriage, they had a lot of sex. Because Mark was in the hospital for a month, and Sue was going to school and working, they had less sex in the first months of their marriage.

During the first five or six years of their marriage, they had problems sexually, and with the relationship in general. They were fighting a lot. They read the books *Loving Relationships* and *I Deserve Love* by Sondra Ray. They called up the Loving Relationships Training office, started getting rebirthed, and took the weekend LRT. Rebirthing and the LRT got them through the rough period of their relationship.

Sue's Personal Lies are THERE IS SOMETHING WRONG WITH ME and I AM NOT GOOD ENOUGH AS A WOMAN. She also feels that I CAN'T DO IT RIGHT AS A WOMAN. Sue's biggest trouble with sex is that she feels she is NOT GOOD ENOUGH WITH SEX and NOT GOOD ENOUGH TO HAVE SEX.

Mark's Personal Lies are I AM NOT GOOD ENOUGH and I AM STUPID. Mark's problem over the years was he thought, I WANT SEX TOO MUCH.

Mark is the initiator in sex. Mark always thought he wanted sex more than Sue. Because Mark felt NOT GOOD ENOUGH, he felt like he did not deserve all the sex he wanted with Sue.

Now, Mark and Sue have sex frequently—three or four times a week. Sex is more playful. In the past, sex seemed more special, and it felt life-threatening if they didn't have sex. Sex is now fun and playful.

Sue loves sex in the afternoons and at unexpected times. She says vacations are always great for her sexually, especially the Ten Day LRT on Physical Immortality. At this workshop in Hawaii, they both received a renewed sense of safety around their sexuality.

Mark feels more comfortable with sex at home than on vacation. He also admits his attraction to good-looking women. He doesn't act out this Suppressed Incest Pattern, but he recognizes and admits it openly now.

Mark and Sue had the following advice for couples in the area of sex and marriage.

1. Let go of the judgements you have about each other.
2. Realize sex goes in cycles. Sometimes you might have a lot of sex and sometimes you might have none.
3. Accept periods of celibacy if they occur in your relationship.
4. Keep sex light and try not to make it too intense.
5. Learn to love affection as well as sex. Women often want affection and not sex.
6. Friendship, communication and fun are the most important ingredients of a good relationship.
7. Similar interests and goals keep people excited about each other.

Sex and Marriage Interview with Tom and Laura

Tom and Laura have been together for nine years. They have been married for four.

They met at a Christmas party. Laura's initial thought about Tom was that he was weird because he said he was God. At the same time she felt there was something to what he was saying. Tom thought he heard celestial music in Laura's presence. His heart chakra opened and he felt that his soul had met a friend.

They started to date after New Year's, when they went to another party at the same house. This party was a costume party.

They started sleeping together almost immediately and Laura got pregnant right away. Tom thought that the sex was magical and intense when they first made love. Laura felt very strong energy in their sexuality together.

Laura was naive before this relationship: she had had very little sexual experience.

Laura had a miscarriage after four months.

In the beginning of their relationship Laura and Tom had sex about three or four times a week. Laura lived one hour away from Tom. She would visit him, spend the night, and they would have sex. They moved in together one year and one day after they started dating. They had been living together for four months when Laura got pregnant again. This was one year after the miscarriage. They thought for two weeks about doing an herbal abortion. They had discord in their relationship even though they were having lots of sex. The sex was intense and good when they moved in together.

Their sexual relationship changed when their child Mark was born. Laura felt that sex went BLAH. She was not as interested in sex as she had been before. Tom took it personally that there wasn't as much sex as before. He felt conflict and competition with his son.

Tom had had a lot of sex with his first wife even after they had children. He was shocked that there was less sex with Laura. Not having sex made him feel inadequate and unwanted by Laura.

Laura's conception was not planned. She was conceived when her brother was two years old and her sister was seven months. Her parents were not ready for her. Her mother thought that sex was a duty. Her mother had been a twin whom nobody knew was in the womb, and therefore she had always felt invisible. Her twin was a male, the wanted one. Consequently Laura's mom used a lot of male energy to try to be more visible and noticed. Her mother always felt that she should not be excited about sex. When she had sex she created having babies she wasn't ready for, just as her parents did not expect her.

Laura feels that she repeats her mother's sexual pattern. She feels that she is not really supposed to be turned on to sex. Her parents had no obvious sexual behavior; they were not affectionate or intimate. She is not affectionate with Tom and often it is hard to tell that they have an intimate relationship. Laura holds back receiving and giving physical affection. Usually she suppresses her sexual, physical energy and doesn't want sex.

In the womb Laura had the thought I AM NOT SUPPOSED TO BE HERE. I SHOULD BE INVISIBLE IN AND OUT OF THE WOMB, SO I DON'T MAKE A PROBLEM. She also has the feeling that she is not supposed to have sex, because that makes her feel too alive. Laura's sister was sixteen months old when Laura was born, and was depressed because she felt replaced by Laura. Laura felt guilty about being alive.

Laura has guilt about her sexual aliveness. She feels that sex and sexual aliveness are bad and dirty. She also feels guilty if and when she receives pleasure. Her mother nursed her but then her mother's nipples cracked and bled. Laura was allergic to non-breast milk so her mother had to breastfeed her even though it was painful. Laura decided that her pleasure caused pain for the ones she loved. She also believes THE PEOPLE I LOVE HAVE TO DO WHAT THEY DON'T WANT TO DO TO GIVE ME PLEASURE.

She received pleasure from masturbating before she knew what she was doing. Her brother also experimented with masturbation and they would talk about it. Her's parents never talked to her about sex—they completely avoided the topic.

Tom's conception was wanted and planned. His trauma was associated with the fact that his parents and older brother wanted a girl. His mother thought that sex was something that you had to tolerate. His dad was an old world Italian. Sexual performance was important. Sex was something you were supposed to do to have children and be a man. In the womb Tom knew his parents wanted a girl. He made the decision that MY SEXUALITY IS WRONG. His brother didn't want him because he didn't want to compete. He was born quickly—in four hours. His mother was heavily anesthetized so she did not support him and she was not there for him. He had a broken collarbone at his birth and he decided that THERE IS SOMETHING WRONG WITH ME.

When Tom was nine, two girls, ages ten and eleven, stroked his penis. He thought it felt great. When he told his mother she told him that sex was ugly, dirty and bad. He is Catholic and the church let him know that sex was bad and created impure touch and thoughts.

Tom's most negative thoughts about sex are:

1. Sex causes pregnancy.

2. There is not enough sex.

3. Sex is confrontive.

Tom's biggest problem with sex is that there is not enough for him. Tom was bottlefed on a schedule. He has the thought that he can't have what he wants when he wants it. Since Tom's Personal Lie is I AM NOT GOOD ENOUGH AS A MAN, he creates not getting enough sex. He feels he really does not deserve the sex he desires. The way Tom wants to improve sex in their relationship is to see that Laura wants sex as much as he does and that she initiates sex.

Laura's three most negative thoughts about sex are:

1. Sex is dirty.

2. Sex is bad.

3. Having sex is too much work.

Laura's biggest problem with sex is that she feels that she is not doing it right, or good enough for the way Tom wants it. Her Personal Lie effects her sexually because she feels bad and guilty for being here and enjoying sex.

Tom says that sex is good when "we are in the flow together and happy, as well as being alive and in sync." Laura says, "Sex is good for us when it is easy and fun. Sex is also good when we are both satisfied and sharing with each other that we are satisfied."

Sex and Marriage

BY BOB AND MALLIE MANDEL

When we got married, we experienced a new state of sexual being. "Virginnocence" we called it, describing the surprising renewal of sexual innocence that entered our lives.

We thought we were fairly well liberated, both spiritually and sexually, before we were married. Certainly, we had no conscious thought of living in sin. We had been together for four years and had fought for our individuality and freedom as forcefully as we persisted in creating our ideal loving relationship. We wanted a holy relationship, but not at the expense of our individual salvation. We were incapable of denying our feelings, so we rode a rocky roller coaster, the destination of which was peace with passion. We re-created, re-lived and released the drama of colliding birth scripts, Personal Lies and family patterns. All the while, our sex life was hot. (Mallie is Scorpio, water. I am Sagittarius, fire. Together, we sizzle.) By the time we had been together four years, we felt we had it pretty much together. Then someone mentioned the dreaded word, "marriage," and suddenly the roller coaster jerked us for another loop.

We began to process our negative thoughts about marriage, knowing that whether we tied the knot or not, we did not want our choice to be in reaction to anything unresolved in either of us. One of our most limiting thoughts was that marriage took the heat out of sex, which was an expression of the deeper thoughts that marriage made life less exciting and eventually killed you. We released these thoughts one by one, as well as many others. On August 6th, 1980 we were married.

Our relationship today is hotter and holier than ever, and we have learned a great deal which we love to share with other couples. Here are some of the lessons:

1. If your sex life is based on performance, conquest and possession, you might have a problem once you are married because then you "have" what you previously were seeking. Once you submit to the mind-set of "having," the part of you that was seeking sexually will lose its passion. The solution is never to think you "have" a relationship. You are in love, which is a continuously transforming and changing state of being. When making love, stay in present time, breathe a lot, surrender to the energy of the moment and let it take you for a ride rather than you trying to control it. We call this "quantum sex" vs. the "linear sex" that tends to focus on performance and conquest.

2. Tell the truth quickly. Before making love, share anything on your minds, positive or negative, that might create distractions from sex. Remember, any withholds from your partner might become energy blocks in your body.

3. Be creative sexually. Sometimes when a couple gets married they unconsciously copy their parents' sexual behavior and fall into a rut. Remember that you are free to play, experiment and explore new ways of connecting physically even though you are married. Marriage is not the end of sexual experimenting, it is the bridge to new creativity. So don't get stuck in one position, as it were.

4. Become more beautiful. Sometimes people let themselves go physically once married. Their attitude is, now that I "have" my mate, I no longer have to struggle to be attractive. Granted, you want to give up the struggle, but not your commitment to your body. If you want great sex in marriage, you must continue to make it a priority to attract your partner. It is your responsibility to create your own beauty. You should have the attitude that you're so attractive your partner can't take his or her eyes off you.

5. Stay seductive. If your seductive energy was based entirely on attracting a mate, once you have your mate, you might unconsciously forget that continuing to seduce him or her is the way to sustain hot sex. Of course, you don't want to go flaunting your seductive energy on others, but it is entirely appropriate to be a turn-on for your mate. Sometimes people unconsciously fall into thinking they can't be sexy in a family, and once you're married you are a new family unit. So you might project your unresolved thoughts and feelings about sex and family onto your marriage. It's okay to have a sexy family.

6. Watch out for time patterns. For example, if your father died when you were three or your parents were divorced when you were five, you

might unconsciously project this separation on your sex life after three, or five, years. Release these past traumas through rebirthing or The Loving Relationships Training or the LRT Couples Retreat.

7. Never take your relationship for granted. Sometimes, when you are secure about the future, you sacrifice the present, whereas when the future is unknown the present is more exciting. Your marriage is not a ticket to the future. It is not a given. It's a process, and the future will always be a result of what you create now. So remember your commitment is to more joy and aliveness now. And the more safety you create physically now, the less security, which is based on fear, will be needed.
8. Plan on sex. You can get so busy with other things in a marriage that you might relegate sex to the back burner, as it were. You might have an aversion to scheduling sex, or scheduling anything for that matter. You might be resentful about having been fed on a schedule, or the schedule surrounding your birth. You might be an unplanned child and therefore think that all planning kills your aliveness. Get through this. You can be in charge of a schedule that supports your aliveness, excitement and sexuality.
9. The honeymoon is never over. This is a very healthy attitude. If the context of your marriage is that it is a continuous honeymoon, an ongoing celebration of your choice to play together, you will naturally have more fun and see your priorities in proper perspective.
10. Remember that your spiritual purpose in being together includes having fun, playing, touching a lot, looking in each other's eyes and experiencing the eternality of your love for each other. The more time you spend practicing your spiritual purpose together, the more you will renew your relationship in a hot and holy energy. Remember, a Holy Instant can be a Sexual Leap as well as a spiritual one. Ultimately, there is no separation between sex and spirit, and the purpose of marriage is to experience sacred sexuality.
11. Don't keep score. Many people have a pattern of keeping score while making love, or in relationships in general, measuring how much they give against how much they receive and having their satisfaction be a result of this equation. This is extremely limiting. Give freely, without obligating your partner. Receive freely, without feeling obligated. A good receiver creates a good giver, and vice versa.
12. Go for quality, not quantity. Quality sex creates sufficient quantity, whereas no quantity is a substitute for quality. Focus on the act of

creation every time you make love, and the love you make will create an abundance of treasured experience in your life.

In the ten years we have been married, we have retained the childlikeness of our sexuality. When we make love, we still feel the "virginnocence" of the experience. And that's how it should be. Because marriage is surrendering your ego's need for separation to a holy union where you have God's permission to have a ball.

So if you approach your sex life with the vigor of a child and the wisdom of an adult, marriage is simply another game in which to express your aliveness fully. Like playing house. You're never too old to play games at home. And sex is just play. It beats the hell out of Trivial Pursuit.

Bob and Mallie Mandel give the 10-day LRT Couples Retreat. If you are interested in finding out about it, contact LRT International, PO Box 1465, Washington, CT 06793. Telephone number 800-INTL-LRT.

Let Go of the Sex Myths In Your Relationship

CONDENSED FROM "FAMILY CIRCLE" BY JANE GASSNER PATRICK

1. Myth: WOMEN ARE LESS INTERESTED IN SEX THAN MEN. This myth is based on the old stereotypes that men are aggressive and women are passive and this is the way it is supposed to be. The truth is, women of good health can have more sexual desire than men. Women are asking for what they want more and more. They are no longer settling for the idea that satisfying men is the duty of women. Women want pleasure too.

2. Myth: THE HARDER YOU FOCUS ON YOUR SEXUAL PERFORMANCE, THE BETTER IT WILL BE. If all your attention is focused on the orgasm you will not feel the pleasure you are receiving in the moment.

3. Myth: SEX GETS BORING WITH THE SAME PARTNER YEAR AFTER YEAR. Being with the same partner allows more intimacy and safety. To maintain freshness, both partners may want to try being more adventuresome, more creative and more playful in their lovemaking.

4. Myth: GOOD SEX HAPPENS WHEN YOU TAKE RESPONSIBILITY FOR YOUR PARTNER'S PLEASURE. During sex it is important to love yourself in the presence of your partner. Great sex comes from knowing what pleases you and taking the initiative to create that happening with your

partner. When your partner is giving to you, let them know what you want and what feels good. When you take responsibility for your own pleasure, this leads to satisfying sex.

5. Myth: MEN HIT THEIR SEXUAL PEAK AT EIGHTEEN AND THEN GO DOWNHILL. Testosterone, the male hormone that influences sexual excitement, is usually at its peak production at eighteen. But a man's sexuality depends on more than physiology. A man having a healthy self-concept and an interested partner can fully enjoy sex indefinitely. The more we focus on our immortality the longer we enjoy our sexual aliveness.
6. Myth: INDEPENDENT, AGGRESSIVE WOMEN MAKE MEN FEEL IMPOTENT. Women do not cause impotence in men. A man's impotence has to do with how he feels about himself and his self-esteem. A woman who is excited about her sexuality and aliveness can inspire her partner to be more alive and sexually active.
7. Myth: SEX SHOULD ALWAYS BE A PASSIONATE, PHYSICAL AND EMOTIONAL COMMUNION BETWEEN TWO PEOPLE. Sex is always unique and different each time you are together. If you try to capture the way sex was in the past, you let the moment go by which could also be a wonderful sexual experience. You distract yourself by having a certain goal in your sexuality. Relax and let go and let yourselves experience where you are with each other in the present moment.
8. Myth: SEX SHOULD ALWAYS BE SPONTANEOUS Many couples are very busy. With both partners working you may find that you are too tired for sex or that you don't have the time to be spontaneous. Schedule special times to be together to be romantic. Don't schedule the sex but schedule the time and place to be together. Then let the intimacy, cuddling, affection and lovemaking happen.

Sex After Sixty

BY GLORIA & JACK LEVAND

(Rhonda's Note: Mom and dad have been married for fifty-eight happy years, and each is seventy-eight years young. They consider themselves Immortalists. They have been very supportive of me, and are LRT graduates.)

With a limited number of words, we will strive to communicate our experiences to Rhonda's readers. However, first, we want to set the record straight about Rhonda's birth. Back in history, we were under age when we eloped to Kentucky in 1932 to get married. While still at Ohio State, we decided to announce our marriage. The announcement coincided with Franklin Delano Roosevelt's closing of all the banks on March 4, 1933. No one gave our marriage more than six months. (Did we fool them!)

In 1935, our first child, Arlene, was born in Columbus, Ohio, and as the Depression disappeared and our income rose, Ellen was born four years later. Then there was a ten-year wait as we built a new home in Cleveland and increased our savings. In 1948, we decided to have one more child—and we did say that we were hoping for a boy to join the two girls. However, we continually told everyone who would listen, "We don't care whether it is a boy or a girl as long as it is healthy".

Each of our children was delivered in our home. When the doctors, Joe and Alex Gross of University Heights, Ohio, eased the baby out of Gloria's womb on March 25, 1949, for a quick instant Jack did display disappointment. But the mood quickly changed to joy and happiness as we welcomed Rhonda into the world. She was the recipient of all the love any parent could give a child, and we still had enough left over so that each child was treated equally with our deep love and affection.

When we were first married, while still in our twenties, like all newlyweds with stars in our eyes, we couldn't get enough sex. Three or four times every night was not unusual. Then, it became twice a week in our thirties, with an occasional morning of lovemaking before breakfast. When we were transferred from Cleveland to Los Angeles we were in our forties, and the move was very traumatic. Psychological problems emerged, and with it a minimizing of sex. All of a sudden we were making love once a week. We called it our "Saturday night special."

Smooth sailing can't always be possible in any marriage, and as a defense mechanism, to erase the pressures, we both began rigid physical fitness programs. Gloria went back into strenuous dance routines, and Jack started to jog, and exercise with weights, after a long layoff from his varsity days at Ohio State. Our diet received a complete overhaul, with natural foods and vitamin supplements. Our menu minimized meat; we only ate what could fly or swim, with lots of fruits and vegetables. Good sex and good physical appearance are synonymous.

In 1962, we began to build our own business, and the struggles in the early stages held down our sex drives. One can see how the mind governs the bedroom. But we resolved to continue to use it so we wouldn't lose it!

Jack did a lot of traveling, and was working long hours in order to assure a good income from his recycling business, Levand Steel & Supply Corp. He augmented his income by becoming a real estate broker. Three girls were assured college educations.

The era of our fifties and sixties were normal for our age group. In 1982, we entered our Golden Age, and began to look seriously at our sexual patterns. Gloria revealed for the first time that somewhere in her fifties, after the start of menopause, that she had hot flashes and a feeling of dryness that adversely affected her sexual pleasures. She said that the juices were not flowing before or during intercourse as they formerly did. We realized that her situation was the equivalent of a man's inability to have an erection. We speculated that this was a result of a loss of estrogen.

We carefully analyzed every aspect of our sexual experience, and recalled the advice of our spiritual advisor who wisely observed: "Sex should be governed by the heart, and not the mind." We then eliminated all the prejudices we had about oral sex, and that resulted in a beautiful reciprocal sex relationship. As we look back, we realize that one must train early for a satisfying lifetime of sexual joy.

Space does not allow for the revelation of little secrets we have for arousal, and other intimate aids for great sex when you are in your seventies and eighties. Briefly, make certain you understand what thrills your partner, and do it! Don't have any inhibitions . . . experiment with different positions . . . have a moonlight dinner with wine . . . . hugs and kisses are important. We are having good sex at least once a week, and plan to continue well up to 100! Great sex is there for you forever, seize it!!!!

Immortal Sex Versus Mortal Sex

Mortal sexuality comes from the ego's thought system. The mortal mind is time-oriented and believes in separation, conflict, fear, pain, anger, worry, misery, scarcity, and depression. When you are in this mind space, your sexuality can only be dissatisfying and frustrating.

Your mortal mind made up your Personal Lie. When you have sex from the mind space of your Personal Lie, you end up feeling more separate from your partner, which creates conflict, and brings fear, pain, anger, worry and misery. Then you usually feel like you will lose your partner, which depresses you.

When you have sex from the mind space of your Eternal Law, you are in your immortal mind, which is timeless. Sex then brings aliveness, love, harmony, peace, safety, certainty, and happiness to the relationship.

A Course in Miracles, Lesson 101, states, "God's will for you is perfect happiness". The more you live in your immortal mind, the more you allow yourself perfect happiness, which is your divine right.

Many people have a lot of guilt about their sexuality. This comes from the ego and the mortal mind. The truth about sex is that it is innocent, and so are you for wanting sexual bliss.

Sexuality is a spiritual act. It is the act of connecting two of God's beings together. In sex, you can become at one, and in tune with another person in a way that is unmatched by any other means of connection. You can become that person, and they can become you. You can merge your minds, bodies and spirits. You can become both male and female. You can blend with another individual, and see and become their perfection.

Being spiritual is recognizing your divinity, as well as the divinity of others. While making love, you have the opportunity to look into the eyes of your partner, past their body and into their soul. You are able to see who they really are, instead of who they pretend to be. You see their beauty, innocence and their Eternal Law. If this isn't spiritual, I don't know what is.

The more I study *A Course In Miracles*, the more I see it as a textbook for sexual bliss. The purpose of the Course is to end separation, to create peace, and the feeling of safety and total trust in our fellow man. Sex is a time to allow surrender, safety and trust into our lives. I notice that the more I connect and let my partner in, the more intimate I become with him. The more I see God in everyone, the more I see the divinity in myself and others.

Allow yourself to experience yourself as a spiritual, sexual being. They are one and the same thing.

Affirmations

1. My sexuality is my spirituality.
2. My spirituality is my sexuality.
3. My sexuality is my divine right.
4. My sexuality is innocent.
5. God approves of my sexuality.
6. I am now willing for my ego to fail, so I can experience sex as totally innocent and divine.
7. Sex strengthens my spiritual bond to God.
8. To receive sexual satisfaction is divine.
9. Thank God for all the sexual pleasure I have.
10. God's will for me is perfect happiness and sexual bliss.

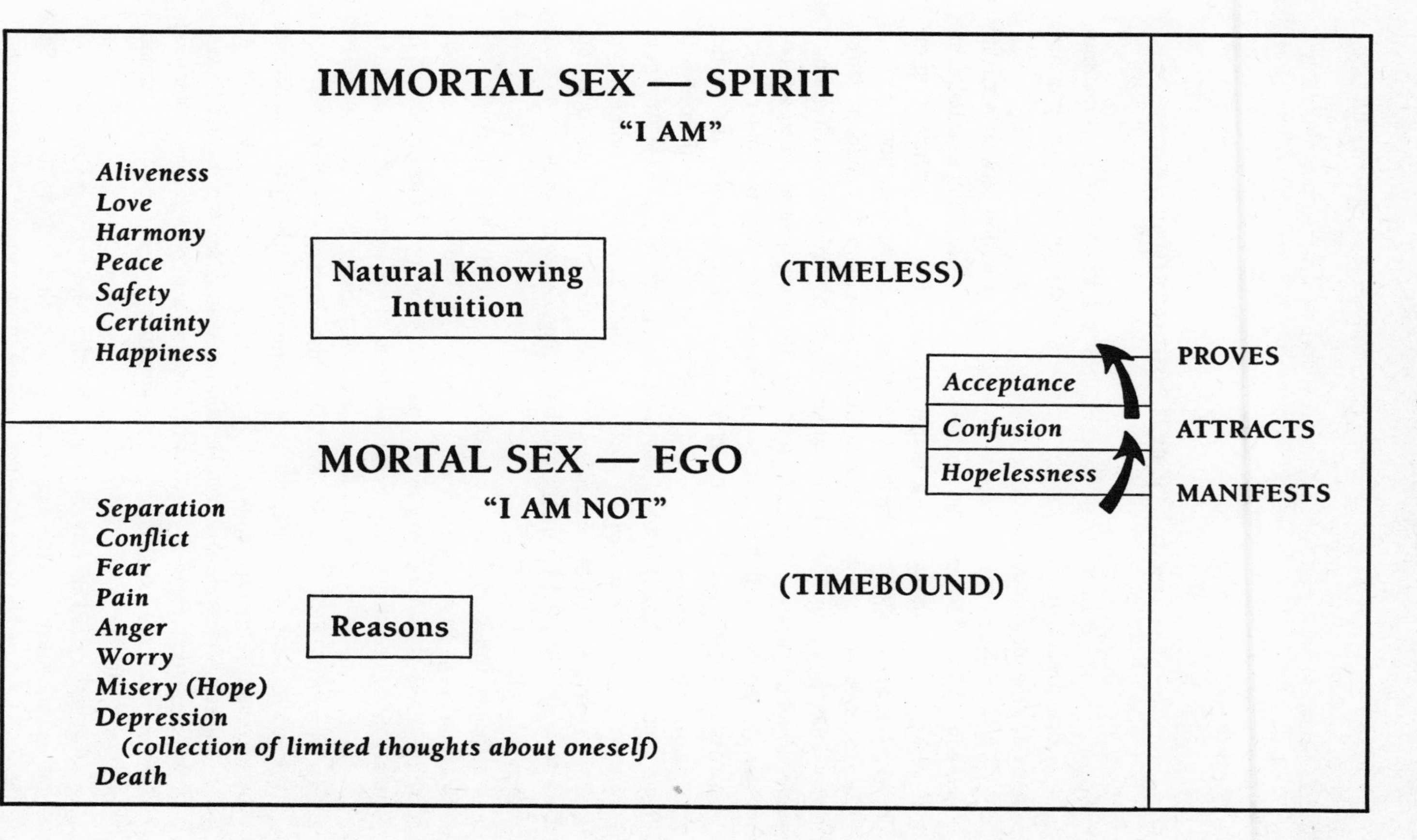
IMMORTAL SEX — SPIRIT
"I AM"
Aliveness
Love
Harmony
Peace
Safety
Certainty
Happiness
Natural Knowing
Intuition
(TIMELESS)
Acceptance
PROVES
Confusion
ATTRACTS
Hopelessness
MANIFESTS
MORTAL SEX — EGO
"I AM NOT"
Separation
Conflict
Fear
Pain
Anger
Worry
Misery (Hope)
Depression
(collection of limited thoughts about oneself)
Death
Reasons
(TIMEBOUND)

11. When I am making love with my partner, I am making love with God.
12. Since I know my sexuality is innocent and safe, having sex affirms my immortality.

Sexuality and Spirituality

Recently, I have returned from my third trip to India. I have been continuously drawn back to India over the past decade, without completely understanding why, until this last trip.

The purpose for me has been to unravel the connection between sexuality and spirituality. These trips have helped me to integrate being a sexual, feminine woman, loving myself as a woman at a deeper level, understanding my own spirituality better, and blending my spirituality and sexuality.

In 1979, I went to India with my first husband and two children. Jarrett was under a year old, and Raynbow was three. My husband Michael and I had a rough marriage—especially sexually. Before we went to India, we took a tantric workshop to heal our sexual issues. The woman trainer was a Rajneesh devotee. This workshop gave us a lot of information, and pushed us through some blocks, but we had not really gotten down to the causes of our problems. I did not know anything about my Personal Lie (my most negative thought about myself), or how my birth and early childhood conditioning had affected my sexuality. We learned a lot of great techniques, but we were unable to follow through with the physical exercises because of our mental blocks.

This course got Michael excited about going to India to study with Bhagwan Shree Rajneesh, who was known for his knowledge of Tantric sexuality. Tantra is learning how to use the sexual energy for enlightenment, or for achieving heightened awareness of God and of the oneness of the universe.

One of my favorite books about sex is Rajneesh's book *Sex*. Often, we have our LIGHTENING UP ON SEX workshop participants read this book as an assignment. There is great wisdom in this book on the connection between spirituality and sexuality.

Rajneesh's message was love. He said celebrating sex is a natural process of transformation. He said, "Sex is to be used as a stepping stone, a stepping stone to move into love, and from love into prayer. Sex is not your creation, but God's gift."

Rajneesh questions you about your beliefs about sex. He asks, "Who told you sex was dirty? All life exists through sex, all life grows out of it. Sex should be a pure phenomenon—two persons in the moment feeling that they would like to communicate on a deeper level. Sex should be playful and prayerful. In sex, there is an alchemical transformation, your woman and man meet inside, and you become one. And when you are one, you will have love."

He also says, "Move into sex consciously! This is the secret to open up a new door." He talks about what an orgasm is, and the difference between an orgasm and just a release of pent-up sexual energy. He asks, "What is Orgasm? Orgasm is a state where your body is no longer felt as matter, it vibrates like energy, electricity. There are no longer boundaries to you. Your frozen energy melts, and becomes one with the universe, and the trees and the stars, and the man and the woman and the rocks—for a single moment. In that moment, you have a kind of consciousness that is religious, that is holy, because it comes from the whole."

Rajneesh states further that, "Without knowing that you can have great orgasmic explosions, you will not be able to understand anything of Spirituality. Orgasm is the meeting of two souls, true orgasm is when you melt into each other. Orgasm is always divine, the other, your partner, becomes the door and you enter the divine. Orgasm is always spiritual. Orgasm is always *samadhi*, ecstasy."

Rajneesh teaches that in order to reach this state of bliss and cosmic orgasm, you have to release all fear of intimacy and closeness. When this state of ecstasy is reached, it is not through goal-oriented sex but through sex that is playful and in the moment.

He also explains, "Sex without love becomes just a trifle. When there is no love the energy moves in a line, a circle of energy is not made. When a circle of energy is created, there you become one. If the circle is total there, both partners will come out of the sex act more energetic, more alive, more changed and with more energy flowing."

Rajneesh describes three elements that must be there to bring you to the blissful moment. "Firstly, Timelessness, you transcend time completely. There is no time. Secondly, in sex for the first time you lose your ego; you become egoless. You and your beloved are lost into something else. Thirdly, in sex you are natural for the first time. You are a part of nature, a part of the trees, a part of the animals, a part of the stars, you are immersed into a greater something, the COSMOS, THE TAO. Your sex energy is your nourishment for your samadhi."

When he talks about *samadhi* he is talking about a blissful state of awareness. He says that by knowing, discovering your sexuality, " . . . one day you will stumble upon your spirituality, and you will then become free."

The main thing I learned from Rajneesh was that suppressing my sexuality also meant I was suppressing my spirituality. The Rajneesh period opened up the beginnings of my sexual-spiritual energy.

Michael, my children and I spent ten days in Poona, India with Rajneesh, in 1979, at his ashram. During this time, we did meditations three times a day: Chaotic meditation, Kundalini meditations, Humming meditations and Dancing meditations. We also listened to his lectures each day. I entered into a state of confusion; my ego and western mind got very confused and started to break down. At that time, I didn't know as I know now that CONFUSION IS A HIGH STATE. Confusion is one of the pathways to the immortal mind, or our deeper connection to God. I felt very separate in the ashram, and I could not wait to get out of there.

During this period, I was reading *Autobiography Of A Yogi* by Yogananda. Babaji was mentioned in this book, and I had a curiosity about him. Someone told us where he was located: outside Delhi in the Himalayan Mountains. We decided to go see him at Herakhan. We had to take mules into the ashram, for there was a four-mile trek down a river bed. When we arrived, it felt like we were in Fantasyland, or at least in another dimension. The ashram was nestled in the mountains, and we had to climb 108 steps to get to it. When we arrived, we saw many people with shaved heads. The first person I saw was wearing a sign saying he was silent for one year, by Babaji's orders. All of this seemed very scary.

That night we had darshan, a meeting with Babaji. He told people how long they could stay. He told many people that they could not stay, and they had to leave immediately. When he got to us, he told us we had no discipline. It was customary to write ahead and get permission to come to the ashram. We had not done this: we had acted spontaneously and just gone there, because on some level we were drawn there. He told us we could stay three days. He let us stay three days mainly because he loved children, and he felt our children needed to rest.

When Babaji told us we had no discipline, it struck my body like a lightning force. I knew he was right; we had no discipline spiritually, mentally, emotionally or physically. It also felt like we had no purpose: we were just moving around the world aimlessly, with no goals or direction. At first, I was disappointed that I could stay only three days. However, at the end of three days we could not wait to get out of there.

Babaji confronted us with all our major issues. It has taken me ten years to integrate and fully understand what happened to me there. Babaji's message is very simple: TRUTH, SIMPLICITY AND LOVE. By repetitively and continuously chanting the mantra, OMNAMAH SHIVAYA, which means "I surrender to the god within," or, "Shiva please destroy my ignorance and ego," you are focusing on God, and expanding the presence of God in your life. There were many ceremonies, and much intimacy, love and deep devotion to Babaji at this ashram. Everything unlike love came up for us; we found ourselves being judgmental, critical and angry, as well as confused.

Babaji was pure, innocent, gentle but firm, and childlike. People would bow down to him and kiss his feet. He might be blowing soap bubbles over their heads. He loved singing and dancing, and he laughed a lot.

Babaji was really processing many of our issues. We had to question our belief in God, our willingness to bow down to him, and all our separation issues. He had us sleeping in the temple, so daily he would process us on how neat we were, or how we had placed our bags. Each day, he would tell us to put our bags a different way. He was teaching our children about discipline and cleanliness. Whenever they wanted something from him, he made them go wash up.

One day, Babaji asked me, "Why are you following this man, when he should be following you?" When he asked me this question, I realized that Michael and I were moving in opposite directions from each other. Rajneesh and Babaji represented two different directions and paths to enlightenment. They represented two different extremes. Rajneesh processed people's egos through confusion. Babaji processed people through discipline, service to mankind through Karma Yoga, and deep love and devotion to God. I seemed to be choosing Babaji's path, though I did not know this at the time, and Michael was choosing Rajneesh's path. Each of these paths fit us, and the other rubbed us the wrong way.

Shortly after we returned from India, I left Michael after seven years of marriage. Babaji brought me to the LRT. I went to a bookstore, and the book *Loving Relationships* fell at my feet. I knew this was something I had to buy. I needed to re-discover who I was and what I wanted to do with my life. I was ready for big changes, and the LOVING RELATIONSHIPS TRAINING provided me with the direction to go that served me the most.

I met Sondra Ray at my first weekend LRT, and she became my pure, spiritual sister, friend and profound teacher. Sondra has been a devotee of Babaji for several years. That's how I know that Babaji brought me to the LRT. The LRT was a more gentle, western way for me to heal myself. I was not quite ready for the eastern way in 1979. The LRT was more compatible with my western mind. Sondra eventually brought me back to India and the eastern way, when I was ready.

My major healing within the LOVING RELATIONSHIPS TRAINING has been of my sexuality and spirituality. Loving myself unconditionally as a woman has been the quest that I have undertaken. I realize now my trips to India have been an integral part of this healing. As I have healed my sexuality, I have also been healing my spiritual connection to God. To become the spiritually enlightened being that I wanted to be, I had to stop suppressing my feminine sexuality. My sexual enlightenment, or LIGHTENING UP, has led to my sexual rebirth and evolution, which at the same time has led to my spiritual rebirth and evolution, my awakening.

In 1985, I went back to India with Sondra and eighty other people, to visit Sai Baba's ashram. The healing I received on this trip was releasing my Personal Lie in relationship to God. My Personal Lie completely separated me from God. Thinking I was a disappointment because I was a woman, and that I was unwanted, wrong, or not good enough because I was a woman, separated me from God, whom I saw as a man. Being a woman separated me from God.

Since I already hated myself as a woman, this gave me more reason to hate being a woman, and also more reason to be angry at God for the separation, and for His being a man. Through Sai Baba, who has very strong feminine energy, and who honored women, I saw that God was also a woman. I instantly felt more connected to God, as well as able to love myself at a deeper level for being a woman.

During a meditation in India, I asked for the discovery and release of any further blocks I had to completely accepting, wanting and loving myself as a woman. I wanted to be strong like a man. I saw that men were the ones that were strong. I injured my eye by scratching it with a metal hairbrush. The eye that I scratched was my left eye, or feminine side. I had been afraid to see my power and strength as a woman. I was blinded to how wonderful it was to be a woman, the creator of life on the planet.

My mother had lost her left eye to cancer. My mother represented to me someone who was not strong: she seemed to depend on my father. I know now that they really depend on each other for different things, and I truly acknowledge my mother's strength. I was into judgement, and did not recognize her strength, or any woman's strength or power. I did not want to surrender to my own divinity as a woman because of my faulty judgements of my mother.

I saw how Sai Baba honored women and the feminine aspect of himself. I then made the turning point in my process of embracing and loving my feminine self, allowing me to love my full and complete self. Because I loved myself at a deeper core level, I was able to surrender to a deeper level of loving God, and recognizing and loving the God in others.

In September, 1989, I returned to India for the third time in a decade, with Jeff, Sondra, and sixty other people. I had another sexual-spiritual healing. Jeff, Sondra, a few other members of the LRT staff, and I, had the wonderful opportunity of living for six days with Shastriji and his family in his home. Shastriji is a saint, and a man of great wisdom. He is the mouthpiece of Babaji, and delivers his messages, as well as doing all the ceremonies during festivals at the ashram. He has written many books.

Jeffrey and I had a reading with Shastriji. He can see the past, present and future in a crystal which Babaji activated for him. One question we asked was if there were anything we needed to heal in our relationship. He told me that I had to let go of my ego, and surrender and follow Jeffrey more. This is the last piece of my sexual issue—surrendering completely to a man in an intimate relationship. This means stop controlling, and let Jeff lead the way.

This is the opposite of what Babaji had told me about Michael. I had been following Michael, and Babaji wondered why. Since that time, I have followed only myself and have never surrendered to following a man. I needed Babaji's permission, in the FORM of Shastriji, to know that it was time to trust and follow a man. Shastriji was letting me know that Jeffrey was the right man to follow, and that I could have more support on my path now. I no longer had to do it alone. Being a strong woman means knowing when to follow and surrender to a man. It is safe for me to follow and surrender to Jeffrey, for he knows the right direction for us now.

I want to acknowledge Shastriji for knowing that I had three more chapters to write for this book. This chapter is extremely important to add in order to pull everything together for me and my own sexual rebirth, as well as for anyone reading this book. After our SEXUAL REBIRTH, we can all experience a new beginning with our Spiritual Awakening.

The last piece of this sexual and spiritual puzzle has to do with Sri Muniraj. Muniraj is Babaji's closest devotee. His name means "King of Sages." Babaji says that Muniraj is no longer bound by the law of birth and rebirth. He is the person in charge of continuing Babaji's work. He was born in Chilyanaula, where we were for the Divine Mother festival. This area is called the Land of the Gods. It is also said that this is where the Divine Mother's home was 20,000 years ago.

Jeffrey and I, Sondra, and the LRT staff members who were there, had a private darshan, or meeting, with Muniraj. At this time, we could ask questions, and be given spiritual names if we wanted them. When I asked Muniraj for my spiritual name, he was silent for a long time. (He is known as the "King of Silence.") He said he was going very deep for my name, and it seemed like forever before he spoke. I am very impatient, and I thought he knew that I was thinking I would never use my spiritual name if he did give it to me. Finally, he told me my name was Radha. I felt the name all through my body, and I felt shivers. Radha is the consort of Krishna, and represents lots of shakti, or sexual energy. I knew the name was perfect for me, based on my sexual-spiritual quest.

Jeffrey was given the name Jai Krishna, which means he embodies all the qualities of Krishna.

I noticed that after we were given our spiritual names, we were drawn to buying silk paintings and statues of Radha and Krishna, which were readily available throughout Delhi. I also bought a beautiful book called *Indian Love*

Paintings by Hilde Bach. Radha and Krishna are on the cover of this book, and throughout the book there are an abundance of pictures of them, and text describing their relationship. When I bought the book I was not aware that one of its central focuses was Krishna and Radha. I have had a very strong attraction to Indian books and the art of India, especially erotic art. One of my favorite books about sexuality is *Sexual Secrets* by Nik Douglas and Penny Slinger. This book talks about Tantric sexuality, and discusses the Indian gods and goddesses, and their influence in the area of sexuality.

I found myself purchasing many statues of Ganesha, the elephant god. I also bought a beautiful, colorful, silk painting of Ganesha, which is hanging beside my two silk paintings of Radha and Krishna in my bedroom. I did not know what my strong attraction to Ganesha was all about, except that I thought he was the god of wisdom, and that he brought prosperity to people. Of course, I wanted prosperity. But I learned he has a deeper significance to me.

I found out from *Sexual Secrets* that Ganesha is considered the embodiment of the Tantric mysteries. The elephant god represents the never-ending storehouse of sexual energy. His trunk symbolizes masculine energy, and his sensuous mouth symbolizes female energy. He is considered the gatekeeper and lord of the sex chakra. His huge strong body and graceful movements represent the mixture of inner strength and sensitivity necessary for spiritual advancement through Tantra.

Ganesha brings good fortune and success to people. Shops throughout India display pictures of Ganesha to guarantee their success and prosperity. Sexual energy is the creative energy which creates good fortune and prosperity. When people open up their sex chakra, wealth and prosperity are increased.

He is also the remover of physical, emotional and psychic obstacles. His name is a powerful mantra, and when it is repeated by someone in difficulty, it will invoke Ganesha's help and support.

Radha, my spiritual namesake, represents success, achievement, and is the presiding goddess of the life energies. She is also a manifestation of Lak Shmi, the goddess of prosperity. I am full of gratitude to Muniraj for giving me this spiritual name, for it is an acknowledgement that I have become the sensual, sexual, prosperous woman I have always wanted to be. Being given this name also means that I am an instrument or vehicle for other women and men to acknowledge their sexuality, and the core of who they really are.

Krishna, Jeffrey's spiritual namesake, is the ideal of the all-potent child, the eternal youth who can take many forms. From the Tantric point of view, Krishna represents the spontaneous power of unconventional love. He represents the embodiment of male eroticism. This makes Jeffrey my perfect compliment and partner. I now see the significance of our workshop, LIGHTENING UP ON SEX, and why we have been placed together to teach this work in the world.

Some quotes from the book *Indian Love Paintings* describe with clarity the connection between spirituality and sexuality.

> "Sex is the supreme fact of life. Sex provides the urge to procreate and maintain the species."
>
> "The sexual Union of Lovers is the most exalted union of lovers in life, and in mutual ecstasy, the liberation of the soul from the narrow 'self' takes place."
>
> "In describing the Union of God and Soul, which many poets and mystics have used to describe 'lover and beloved' (Radha and Krishna), it is seen that Spiritual Love has its roots in Physical Love."
>
> "Love is a gift of one to the other, in which the EGO disappears when the sentiment of love takes possession of the body and soul of the persons in love, this results in companionship and deep intimacy."
>
> "One loves not with just the body. It is when the body and mind are entirely engrossed in another person that one reaches the joyous state of selflessness."
>
> "The love of Radha and Krishna symbolizes the love of the soul for God, personified in Krishna, Krishna represents the soul's search to escape the allurement of the senses, and to find peace in the mystical union with God."
>
> "Krishna and Radha are depicted as ideal lovers. The true relationship of the devotee to God."
>
> "The love of Krishna and Radha is the absolute, self-surrender of the human soul in Radha to the Divine in Krishna is summed up as all love."
>
> "Krishna and Radha's love represents when the finite is brought into the presence of the infinite. The consciousness of inner and outer is destroyed in the ecstasy of union with one beloved."

The message of Indian art and literature is that human love and its physical, sexual expressions are pure, innocent, spiritual, holy and beautiful. In the ecstasy of human love, we experience a glimpse of a greater, more encompassing love that binds the universe together, THE LOVE OF GOD. The unity of two lovers in ecstasy creates two beings egoless in their God State.

In *Sexual Secrets,* Shan Ku San Tai says, "The union of man and woman is like the mating of HEAVEN AND EARTH. It is because of their correct mating that Heaven and Earth last forever. Humans have lost this secret, and have therefore become mortal. By knowing this secret, the path to immortality is opened."

If this section has created curiosity in you about India, Sondra Ray leads the India Quest every year at the time of the fall Divine Mother's festival, in September or October. If you would like information about this spiritual quest, contact LRT International, PO Box 1465, Washington, CT 06793. Telephone number, 800-INTL-LRT.

Lightening Up on Sex

Jeff and I have done LIGHTENING UP ON SEX weekends throughout the world. The participants in those weekends provided the case histories for this book, and many of the processes in the book are used in the weekends.

We are all far too serious about sex. We have found that talking a lot about sex with a group of people releases the pressures and demands we sometimes feel about our sex lives. We have fun doing this workshop, using humor to move ourselves and others through sexual issues and fears of intimacy.

In the workshops, people find they are not alone with their feelings and hangups about sexuality. This usually makes people feel better—misery loves company—to know that they are not the only ones who have issues about sex. The group is also a great support system. All the energy and love exuded from a group helps to push things up and out faster.

Also, men and women get a better understanding about each other's vulnerabilities and needs. They begin to dissolve their differences, and see and understand their similarities. We all want love, peace, prosperity, happiness and sexual bliss.

Sexual issues are universal. The same issues come up for healing in Europe, Australia, New Zealand and the United States. We all need to celebrate our similarities, and dissolve our differences.

If you have enjoyed this book and received value from the information, you might want to go through the experiential part of dealing with your sexual issues by taking a seminar.

If you have never taken the Loving Relationships Training (LRT), know that it is a wonderful way to begin to experience the safety of a group process for self-improvement. Books give you great mental realizations, and rebirthing and seminars support you in releasing the past, and integrating the new information into your body.

Once you have taken the LRT, LIGHTENING UP ON SEX is a fun, easy way to focus on your relationship with your sexuality. What you focus on expands, so if you focus for a whole weekend on having a great sexual relationship, ultimately that will be the result.

For information about LIGHTENING UP ON SEX workshops throughout the world, call (404) 977-3043 or write: Rhonda Levand, 3770 Greenview Ave., Marietta, GA 30068, or contact LRT International, P.O. Box 1465, Washington, CT 06793, phone (800)-INTL-LRT.

CHAPTER 7

Sexual Case Histories

THE FULL SEXUAL case histories in this chapter are good examples of how conception, birth and early childhood affect our sexuality.

These case histories were written as assignments in LIGHTENING UP ON SEX weekends and 10 Day Rebirthing Trainings, in the United States and abroad. People were asked to reveal a lot about who they were and what made them click sexually.

In case you would like to write your own sexual history in order to get a deeper understanding of yourself, the following is a list of what should be included:

1. Conception description.
2. How your conception affects your sexuality.
3. Birth description.
4. How your birth affects your sexuality.
5. Your Personal Lie, or your most negative thought about yourself.
6. How your Personal Lie affects your sexuality.
7. Your biggest problem with sex.
8. How your Personal Lie affects your biggest problem with sex.
9. Childhood incidents of sexuality, ages four to six.
10. Puberty incidents of sexuality, ages eleven to fourteen.
11. Masturbation: when you started and your feelings about it.
12. Your most embarrassing sexual situation.

13. Describe your first sexual experience.

14. Church conditioning about sex.

15. Parental conditioning about sex.

After reading the sexual histories, you might feel inspired to write your own. You will discover how much one's sexuality is influenced and conditioned by one's conception, womb time, birth, and first five years of life.

Sexual Case Histories

1. Ola—Wanted; easy birth.
2. Jane—Planned; wanted; induced.
3. Kathy—Wanted; parents drunk at conception; drugs.
4. Tonya—Wanted and planned; hurry up and wait birth.
5. Steve—Wanted and planned; wrong sex; forceps; incubator.
6. Susan—Unplanned; two weeks premature.
7. Don—Unwanted; jaundiced at birth.
8. Bert—Parents not ready; he was a burden; easy birth.
9. Tom—Unwanted; not born when he wanted to be.
10. James—Unwanted by dad; RH transfusion.
11. Evelyn—Unwanted; hurt at birth.
12. Daniel—Parents not ready; fast birth.
13. Arnette—Illegitimate; mother loved another man.
14. Theresa—Illegitimate; late; mother hurt at birth.
15. Chris—Unwanted; father had affairs; induced.
16. Nancy—Unwanted; easy birth; drugs.
17. Marybeth—Unwanted; three weeks late.
18. Linda—Wrong sex.
19. Debi—Wrong sex; held back; drugged; cord around neck.
20. Joy—Wrong sex; premature; three weeks in incubator.

21. Diana—Wrong sex; forceps; long labor; needed to be turned.
22. Patty—Wrong sex; long separation from mom; two weeks in hospital.
23. Sally—Wrong sex; induced.
24. Connie—Wrong sex; cord around neck; drugs; held back; acted-out incest.
25. Sue—Wrong sex; caesarean; long labor; drugs; separation.
26. Lois—Wrong sex; face presentation.
27. Glenda—Wrong sex; forceps; drugs.
28. Gary—Forceps.
29. Diane—Fast birth; held back; drugs.
30. Eve—Anger at conception; separation at birth.
31. Briar—Wanted to replace sister who died; late birth; fast and easy birth.
32. Alison—Unwanted; three weeks late; dry birth.
33. Robert—Unwanted; drugs; caesarean.
34. Joe—Breech; late birth.
35. Charleen—Forceps.

1. OLA

Conception description .... My mom and dad rode together on their motorcycle and had lots of fun together. (I rode in mom's belly up to the ninth month—today I love motorcycles!) Mom and Dad had good sex together. I was wanted. It had been four years since my sister was born. I was Dad's favorite.

How my conception affects my sexuality .... I too enjoy sex a lot. No hang ups. Dad was partial to girls, especially to me. I was his favorite—I looked like him and his aunt. I copied myself after him—I was told I won a beauty contest as the most beautiful baby. I have always felt beautiful and attractive to men. I liked this, but was unsure how to act around men, and was very naive. I fell for flattery—played right into it. I had an easy birth, I was told. Little chloroform. No problems.

My Personal Lie is .... I CAN'T DO IT GOOD ENOUGH.

How my Personal Lie affects my sexuality .... I can't do it good enough. I'm weak and helpless. I almost never initiate sex or advances, occasionally I will shyly. I thought "I can't do it good enough" until I was excellent at it—I read lots of books. Even "Reader's Digest" articles. I got better and better. Sex is still my greatest fun, my greatest tranquilizer.

I had six children. I tried everything for birth control. I loved being pregnant. I wanted to stop after four (for a rest). I wanted to stop very badly after five. I found the IUD after six.

My biggest problem with sex and my Personal Lie .... I can't do birth control good enough. I tried everything. I became a nurse and my husband was a pharmacist. I kept getting pregnant. I am a weak, helpless, undisciplined child.

Childhood incident of sexuality .... My first experience as a child was with my brother and friends. We looked at each other and played doctor.

Church conditioning .... They never mentioned sex. (They would have said no sex until marriage.)

Parental conditioning .... I left home to go to nurses' training. My mom said, "I hope you don't have to be married, like your sister." Nothing else ever said.

Masturbation .... I masturbated quite a lot. I felt guilty because I was caught once and spanked by my mom at age six or seven. Once I was baby sitting and did something to a two-year-old boy—but I never ever spanked my six kids.

2. JANE

Conception description .... My parents wanted children. My mother had been ill with tuberculosis (caught whilst she was a student nurse) before they married, and they had to wait eighteen months for permission from her doctors before they could try for a baby. My father is thirteen and a half years older than my mother: he was 39, she 25. She was in a power struggle with his mother, who lived just down the street, and who seemed to come first with my father. It was six months before they conceived, and my mother was beginning to worry that she couldn't conceive, like her mother, who was married sixteen years before she conceived.

I feel there was lots invested in my conception; many expectations. I was the first grandchild (and the only prospect of one) for both sides of the family. I think my mother also thought a child would confirm her status. She was seen by everyone as young, rather helpless, or foolish and childlike. She felt like an outsider, coming into my father's social circle. I feel my father had some fear of intimacy.

How my conception affects my sexuality .... I have had the thought "I can't" and fear of failure or being a disappointment a lot in relationships. Also, I realize that I waited for permission until a few years ago before I experimented with masturbation (I read a book that recommended it for premenstrual tension).

Birth description .... "I can't" and "I'm a disappointment" were re-inforced at birth. My father's mother died when I was due, so I arrived eleven days late into a family focused on her death.

My mother was in labor for 48 hours in all; I was induced after 36 hours, because the doctor was worried that she was exhausted. She felt she couldn't push because she had weak stomach muscles. She was encouraged to sleep as much as possible during the labor.

My father was at home; he turned up an hour after I was born, upsetting my mother and explaining why he couldn't stay long, rather than wanting to see me straight away. Mother and I stayed in the hospital a fourth night so she could rest; meanwhile my father's sister had moved in and stayed for eighteen months. She and my mother battled over who came first with my father and whose baby I really was!

How my birth affects my sexuality .... Some of the negative thoughts I have that relate to my sexuality are: "My aliveness is too much or inappropriate", "I can't have what I want", "Everyone else is involved in a drama that I'm outside of and don't understand", "I'm not good enough", "I'm a disappointment", "I have to survive on my own". In some weird way, I even feel responsible for my grandmother's death, or that I was supposed to take over from her or compensate for her loss.

Parental conditioning .... My parents have always shown physical affection for each other, and it's obvious their sex life is a way they show their love. They are both into family tradition, especially my father. I was told always that our family marries late (my father was 39; grandmother 31; aunt 56).

These were the three people I was supposed to take after. They also hold out for the one and only perfect partner. I saw my parents' relationship as unequal: my father had all the power and authority and came first always, my mother was portrayed by him as foolish and childlike and helpless.

My mother impressed on me that to deserve a relationship I must be self-sacrificing, put myself second to my man, and definitely not be intellectual or aggressive or independent. My feelings about this were that I simply could not be the person she wanted me to be, even if it meant being alone. There was also sibling rivalry with my younger brother—whatever he was, I couldn't be, and vice versa. He was charming, attractive, outgoing and like our mother.

Church conditioning . . . . We were with the Church of England and took religion seriously. I think the main ideas about sex I picked up from the Church were that real, full human beings were men, like God was a man, and women's sexuality was evil and low—a snare and a delusion. To be spiritually acceptable you should be celibate and hold out for the one and only. Confirmation classes when I was fourteen stressed that sex was a heavy responsibility with dire consequences, and that it's always the woman's fault, because she leads the man on.

Puberty . . . . I went to a girls' school and a women's college. Even in junior school, boys and girls were not allowed to play together. I used to get really annoyed. I wanted to be friends with boys. As a teenager, my only opportunity to meet boys was at the occasional disco (I grew up in a small country town). I hated the instant groping, but I thought I was unreasonable wanting to be friends first, so I tended to shut off entirely. I felt outside the game everyone else was involved in—I didn't "fancy" every boy as the other girls seemed to. I was also far taller than most of the boys, overweight and short-sighted. In short, I felt humiliated, rejected, resentful and angry.

Sexual experience . . . . My situation is that I am thirty-one and still a virgin. Until a few months ago I had never even kissed a man, let alone gone out with anyone or formed any kind of relationship. The older I got, the more impossible it seemed to begin—I felt extremely foolish and self-conscious. Before I started rebirthing, I had suppressed all my feelings about this so that I rarely saw any man as attractive. I believed there was something wrong with me at a deep level that meant I wasn't capable of having a relationship, and I refused to allow myself to feel sad about it. I tried to make myself believe there was no way out, that I had to be alone. I think becoming thirty shook me up. Anyway, I succeeded in making myself feel light-headed and queasy all the time, and got into rebirthing in an attempt to feel well again. (It worked, naturally.)

Very few men ever actually wanted to go out with me, and never anyone I felt attracted to. I was deep into the "worthless shit syndrome". There was one occasion that really embarrassed me, when someone I'd known at university sent me a beautiful water color he'd done for me with a joking caption underneath. I sent him a postcard thanking him, and it wasn't until I saw him weeks later, and he asked me if I'd liked what he'd written on the back, that I realized there was a love poem on the other side!

My one sexual experience so far was an experience a few months ago with a friend. We were both clear this was strictly a one-night stand (I blame it on my rebirther, who had me affirm "It's safe and OK for me to have casual sex now.") We had no contraceptives, so we stopped short of actual intercourse. It was great to discover I actually enjoyed the whole thing—I'd thought I'd be revolted by it. It was fun and easy and pleasant, but I decided the next time I want to have it all, and experiment within a loving relationship.

I'm working with my fear of intimacy and the feeling that I have to be alone to survive. Also with the thoughts that what I want is unreasonable, and I don't deserve it.

3. KATHY

My conception was .... My guess is that my parents were probably loaded and just having a good time. My dad said Mom wanted children, and the idea was OK by him too. My father said my mother wasn't much for sex until they met. He said they usually had a good time. Nothing fancy, but good. (He was usually pretty out of it as he was into drinking and drugs. They were divorced when I was eighteen months old because he was irresponsible. I guess they started fighting a lot, drinking and doing drugs).

He also said that after they got divorced, other men would call him and ask if there was something wrong, as they couldn't get close to mom physically. My thought about this is that they just were not the right ones. (I remember most of the men around, and they were more like the fatherly type.) She didn't want to make another mistake. Also, she was afraid of sex and felt guilty about it. She died at 42 from cancer of the female organs. She was into metaphysics, but I don't thing she could let go of her fear and guilt. (My father was her second husband. She had no previous children and was not married very long the first time.) Men used to shower her with gifts, and take her out, and be very nice to me.

How my conception affects my sexuality .... In most of the sexual relationships I had before I got married, I was always loaded. I usually had a good time sexually—a pretty wild time. I always considered myself a fairly attractive woman (when I am thin), but all the men I was really interested in always left or were irresponsible. With my husband, our sexual relations were usually when we were loaded. He was very much like what I would guess my father was like when Mom met him. In his own world, hearing only what he wanted to hear—forgetful, confused, caring and soft. Our sex life was great.

My thought is that people who love me, leave me because I'm not good enough. I am also always trying to fix everything. Maybe my mom thought that after I was born, things would straighten out, that my presence would heal their relationship. Maybe Dad would become responsible and stop the drinking and drugs. He didn't. "I'm not good enough to fix it, (their relationship)."

Description of my birth .... My mother died when I was twelve, and my father is an alcoholic (sober for eighteen years now). Dad doesn't remember much of what happened during his drinking years, but what he does remember is that he was working, and came home to get Mom when she went into labor, and took her to the hospital. This was in the afternoon, and I was born at 7:00 in the morning. (I'm sure Mom had some kind of drugs—I'm just not sure what.) My guess is it was a long labor and a bit difficult. When Dad went in just after I was born, Mom was awake and coherent, and I was in the room with them. Her words to Dad were, "No wonder I had such terrible heart burn, look at all that hair!" I think both of my parents had good senses of humor.

How my birth affects my sexuality .... I feel I have to work long and hard, like my mother's labor, and be very patient, in order to fix things and receive love.

My memories of my first sexual feelings .... I was about five years old when Brian moved into the neighborhood. He was about eight years old—a child actor. My best friend and I would play "dreamer" with Brian. He would sit in a lawn chair, close his eyes, and pretend to fall asleep. Then he would sleep walk and marry one of us. He'd put his arm around us and kiss us. It always made me feel important and loved. My best and very first friend and I were both from divorced families living with our moms. Brian's dreams were very important to both of us. (No judgements or negative thoughts, as our parents were never around, and if they were, they thought it was cute.)

Besides Brian my interests leaned more towards the girls. At five, a girl neighbor used to ask me to give her backrubs and touch her breasts on the side. She would giggle and I would get very turned on. I always loved to look and touch my friends bodies—both boys and girls.

I also remember mom was dating an older producer—just friends—no sex. They used to leave me at his house to watch a big T.V. alone when they went to screenings. He had a lot of Playboy magazines, so when they went out I would look at them and get turned on. I used to look forward to going there to look at the books. At some point, he started hiding them. My thought was, "Men don't want me to have pleasure".

My first sexual experience, in puberty .... At age fourteen or fifteen, I was at a pretty risky party (junior high), and this good-looking fellow (a lot of the girls chased after him), ended up with me. A bunch of kids were making out in the driveway—a lot of passionate kissing and touching. He had his hand down my pants and inside me. I put my hand down his pants and felt something very hot and big. I came immediately.

The first time I had intercourse .... I was sixteen—with my boyfriend of about four months. Two of my girlfriends (who are now gay), my boyfriend and I, had gone down to the beach at night during a big fire in a major canyon. The sky was all lit up like a red fireworks display. The winds were blowing strong, and the weather was hot. My two friends went to run on the beach. Ken and I stayed in the van—he promised he would be gentle, and pull out before he came, and he did. Right in the middle of it, my two friends came back and started rocking the van and carrying on. We were all laughing.

My thought then was, "I'd rather be with the girls". They were having fun and I really wasn't. Approval from girls was real important. The experience wasn't too bad. It hurt a little, but by no means was it sexy or passionate. About two or three weeks later, he came over and informed me I needed to be checked for V.D. That was in my father's drinking days. My father threatened Ken, and a few months later he was out of my life. I was heart-broken.

All the men in my life have either had very feminine tendencies (some had relationships with men), or they were still in love with other women who had left them. I have had a lot of mental abuse, and in one case physical abuse, with my partners. Or they have been into drugs and alcohol. Usually they have had a combination of the above conditions. It has been a very 50/50 situation as to who would leave whom. They have all been good looking.

The thought I usually had when they left me was, "I'm not good enough to have a handsome man who has money and love. I'm not good enough to have it all." The thought I had when I left them was, "I deserve a man with more ambition, and no drug and drinking problems." I also loved to do drugs and drink, but I usually kept it together and didn't get ugly and nasty—most people didn't know when I was loaded. I am sure this is how my mother felt about my dad, and why she left him.

Mom and Dad were divorced when I was eighteen months old. I remember always being surrounded by women. My mom was a make-up artist, and worked around a lot of models and gay men designers. I didn't have much of a masculine figure to grab on to. We always had single women roommates with kids and most of my mother's friends were single with kids, so it really was very natural for there not to be a man around. My father came back into my life around age nine.

At seven, my best friend and I created being molested by a Mexican man. I was lucky—I was wearing tights and all he did was grab me in the crotch a few times. As I recall, he did more to my friend, although I didn't see it. We decided that it was funny. But we had to go choose him from a line-up, and go to court, as he had raped several other women. It was a big case!

It happened during the period when my dad was gone. I remember the police car picked me up at school and took me to the station to pick the man from the line-up. My mother wasn't available to go with me and I was very scared. My thought was "No one is there for me, I have to do it myself".

That night my mom said to me, "Are you sure you chose the right man?" I said, "Yes!" She kept asking me over and over. Then she said, "It could be someone else's dad, and you don't want to send an innocent person to jail." But I interpreted it as, "He's probably going to go to jail for a long time, and that could be your dad."

My dad was in prison at this time for an attempted robbery with a toy gun, in one of his drunken stupers. He confessed this to me after my first LRT, when I was 28. My thoughts about men were, "Men do bad things. You can't trust them. I'm afraid of them. They are liars and irresponsible."

Since my mother was always busy and had very little time for me, I thought, "Everyone else is more important than me." I always had the thought that my mother always left me. She truly proved it when she died. (What little time we did share I remember as touching and loving.) When my mom died, I moved in with my dad and his new wife. He was still drinking, so he confirmed all my thoughts about men.

Since Mom abandoned me and Dad was irresponsible, I had to learn how to survive on my own. No one really loves me. No one shows me love. (Everyone loved to have me around, but no one really showed me love.) At around seventeen, I fell in love with a good friend (female), who I'm sure had the same thoughts: "No one really loves me." "No one shows me love." We discussed some of the feelings we had for each other together. She started having sexual relations with other women. When I confronted her, she asked if she could kiss me—I melted and so did she. It never went any further—I tried in subtle ways to be closer to her, but she had a wall up. I did, however, have sexual relationships with other women. I'm sure I was looking for what I felt I was cheated out of by my mother.

Masturbation . . . . For as long as I can remember it has been very easy for me to get turned on. I could get creamy pants looking at books and doing what I've come to know as kegel exercises. I don't actually remember touching myself until around sixteen or so.

One of my mother's previous roommates gave me a book called *The Hite Report,* and told me it was a must to read. We were on vacation. I started reading the chapter on masturbation—it was the first time I had heard about it. The book said there was nothing wrong with it, so I tried it that night and loved the feeling. My biggest concern was I that I would break out if I did it to often. There must have been a story in the book with reference to that fear. When I think of a woman masturbating it seems sensuous, but when I think of a man doing it, it seems dirty. (Maybe because it's messy.)

My biggest problem with sex now is . . . . I feel like I'm under a lot of stress. When my husband and I first got together I wasn't working. He was in the music business, so when he was home he had lots of time too! Our sex life was great! Very intimate and passionate. We spent lots of time together.

His wife had died in the past year and he was in mourning when we met. I think he felt guilty about having feelings for me so soon after her death. Six months after we started spending so much time together, he chose to move away. "I'm not good enough to fix things and receive love." When he moved away, he didn't call me, I had to call him. I saw him maybe two times in the next six months. He suggested I go out with other men. He had also told me that he couldn't feel love again after his wife.

I started dating again and was just starting to move on with my life, when a call came from my husband saying he was going back on the road, and what did I think? I asked him why he was asking me. He then explained that he would need to stay at my place during rehearsals, and that he wanted to take me to Hawaii in August after the tour. I was very angry, and felt guilty that I had been with other men. I ended up creating an abnormal cell growth on my pap smear. He flew home the weekend I had what they called a cervical freeze. He was very sweet and romantic. While he was on the road he had slept with someone else too. I felt it and confronted him. At first he denied it, then he confessed. Our sex life and relationship never regained the intimacy and passion it once had.

Now I have created my daughter being sick most of the time—chronic croup, sinus and ear problems, and money being scarce—no extra, just enough to get by. My husband works nights, and the only time we really have alone together is Sunday night. We don't always make it to the bedroom together on that night either. Both of us are pretty tired and stressed, keeping it together. I met my husband when he was 36. Six years later our daughter was born when he was 42. This is the same age as my mother was when she died.

When I married my husband I married:

My father in his drinking days	• irresponsible • forgetful • selective memory • loving, caring, warm, soft • same astrological sign
My best friend from elementary, jr. high school, and high school	• moody!!! • extremely sensitive!!! • physically strong • sensuous • good looking • good body • angry • selective hearing • stubborn • same astrological sign
My stepmother disapproval	• wants me to be wrong • mis-directed anger • right and wrong is very important

I am ready to have the intimacy and passion back in my relationship, my family to be healthy, and to have lots of money. I'M GOOD ENOUGH TO HAVE IT ALL!!!!

4. TONYA

Conception description . . . . I was a planned baby girl by both my mother and daddy. They wanted a girl. In fact, my parents used a vinegar solution to change the ph in the uterus combined with temperature and timing! I'm very much wanted!

How my conception affects my sexuality .... Sometimes I want to plan a very sexy and romantic evening—to take charge.

Birth description .... Hurry up and wait. I was born between 1 and 2 a.m.

How my birth affects my sexuality .... I never feel as though I could hurry and have an orgasm! I enjoy making love on a cold day under lots of blankets! On an average evening or morning of making love, it seems my extremities are always cold (maybe cause I'm wearing little teddies or hardly anything). Then after coming, I have to be wrapped up under blankets! I prefer to make love in the morning. I seem to be more alive, responsive and downright horny!

My Personal Lie is .... I AM GUILTY.

How my Personal Lie effects my sexuality .... If my husband happens to be horny and I'm not, I feel very guilty! I have felt extremely guilty for having sex before I was married—then I got pregnant and had an abortion! When I was in high school and dating I was a prick tease, but mainly because I wouldn't have sex, this made me feel guilty at times! I had a thought that either I should have sex, or just not date. In college, at seventeen, I had sex for the first time. I caught gonerrhea and got pregnant. We were going to get married, but then I decided I didn't want to get married just because I was pregnant!

My biggest problem with sex is .... If both my husband and I don't come, I feel guilty! If we don't have sex often I feel guilty. It takes a lot of time—45 minutes to two hours.

Affirmation .... We always come at the right time.

5. STEVE

Conception description .... I was planned and wanted. I think my parents were very conscious of the possibility of becoming pregnant. The pregnancy validated their sexuality.

How my conception affects my sexuality .... When I have sex, I am real conscious of not wanting pregnancy. I feel guilty for having sex without the intention of getting pregnant.

Birth description . . . . I was a forceps birth. I felt smothered at my birth. I was not nursed, and put in an incubator. My parents wanted a girl because they had a boy already—this was a disappointment. After birth, I was kept in a playpen separate from my parents.

How my birth affects my sexuality . . . . I resent being controlled in sex. I am not attracted to large breasts because they smother me. I can't have what I want sexually. I continue to isolate and keep myself separate from my partner. My parents thought I was the "prettiest" of the four boys, and often they introduced me as their little girl. I had incest with my oldest brother and always took the female role.

In high school, I went through a period where I was persecuted by the other boys because they thought I was gay. In my twenties, I explored the gay community to resolve my own sexual identity. Today, I am not turned on at all by men, and I am very turned on by women. I like to look at female pornography, but I also use dildos anally while I masturbate.

My Personal Lie is . . . . I AM WRONG AND UNWANTED AS A MAN.

How my Personal Lie affects my sexuality . . . . I have the thought that what I want sexually is wrong, and that I will be rejected or unwanted for it. Basically, the same events and thoughts that led me to form my Personal Lie have continued to prove themselves in my sex life as in all areas of my life.

My earliest memories of my sexuality . . . . When I was four and five, at night, in the closet, my brother and I sucked each other off.

Church conditioning . . . . Dad was the music leader. Every time the church door opened, I was reminded that sex was ultimately wrong unless you were married, and then it was only for having kids.

Parental conditioning . . . . My parents told me all the technical and moral information. There was a lot I missed about emotions and innocence.

My most embarrassing situation . . . . Was being caught in the act by the police when having sex with a girlfriend.

Childhood incidents . . . . I had a full sexual relationship with my older brother for approximately ten years throughout my childhood. We tried to get our two younger twin brothers involved also, but they were not interested. My brother was two years older than me. We started with oral sex, and consummated shortly thereafter with anal intercourse. The first couple of times it was incredibly painful, but I was persuaded to try it again until I started to like it. I usually took the female role, and I came to want it at least as much as he did. Often I wanted it more than he did.

This relationship continued throughout childhood and half way into high school. It stopped when my brother got involved with girls. There were times that we had sex two or three times a week. Then there were other times when we might go months without having sex. We were always very close—he was my best friend. We got into drugs together, about the same time that we stopped having sex with each other. Our relationship started to deteriorate after the drug period.

6. SUSAN

Conception description . . . . I don't really know about my conception, but intuitively I feel it was awkward and not planned.

Birth description . . . . I was born about two weeks early, under anesthesia, after being rushed to the hospital. I was underweight, and placed in an incubator for eighteen days. My mother didn't see me until the eighth day, and she was afraid of me when I went home. I was so small, she thought she'd hurt me.

How my birth and conception affect my sexuality . . . . I feel awkward sometimes having sex. I am also reluctant to be touched a lot. Sometimes I feel I never developed physically as a woman, and my body was always protected and de-emphasized.

Childhood incident of sexuality . . . . I was sitting on the lap of an older cousin—he had an erection and started joking about it. It freaked me out, and I got down off his lap in confusion. I felt it was wrong, even though there was also the thought that it was fun.

My first sexual experience . . . . My first marriage was at the age of twenty-one. The wedding night, after a four-year courtship and doing everything sexually except having intercourse, was very painful. My husband couldn't penetrate my hymen. I went to a doctor the next day to break it. It was weird. Sex in this marriage never really got anywhere. I was always afraid of getting pregnant, and never was turned on by this man.

Church conditioning . . . . Catholic—no sex before marriage—sex is only to have children (and since I never wanted children, I never wanted sex). Also masturbation was a sin, and since I did masturbate at an early age, I was always confessing this "bad" thing I'd done.

Embarrassing situation around sex . . . . When my first husband and I had a somewhat "open" marriage, there was a man I was attracted to, and we tried to have intercourse in a hammock (we were in Mexico). It didn't work! He was gigantic, and it freaked me out, I was shocked that there was such an attraction, and then it had an abrupt end.

My Personal Lie is . . . . I'M WRONG AS A WOMAN.

How my Personal Lie affects my sexuality . . . I play down being a woman. I thought it would make sex better that I couldn't have children—I had a tubal ligation at age 26. I don't like make-up, jewelry, clothes—what most women seem to like.

7. DON

Conception description . . . . My mother stayed with my dad three years more than she wanted to because she got pregnant with me.

How my conception affects my sexuality . . . . I often think a woman will lose out if she loves me. I resist receiving her love because I think she loses if I gain. I often feel unworthy of really receiving.

Birth description . . . . I know I was born with some jaundice, and had blood tests every four hours for a couple of days. I fought getting my foot poked with the needle.

How my birth affects my sexuality . . . . My basic underlying fear is that women will reject me because I'm not good enough.

My Personal Lie . . . . I'M NOT GOOD ENOUGH, I AM UNWORTHY.

How my Personal Lie affects my sexuality . . . . In late elementary school and high school I was a typical horny adolescent, but I had no social graces. I was a nerd.

Circumcision .... My dad took me to be circumcised when I was six months old. I had some complications with my penis when I was four. Since then, I have had fantasies of torturing, mutilating genitals, and raping. The rape fantasies also tie in with wanting to dominate, to be powerful. If I'm afraid of getting rejected or not being good enough ... "Well fuck you! I'm going to just take what I want!"

The last few months I have had an irritation on my penis, probably right where my foreskin used to be. I irritate it when I masturbate, and then I get to feel guilty about masturbating. It's also a good excuse to avoid seeking sex.

Early embarrassing situation .... In sixth grade, I wrote a love note and gave it and a toy ring to a fifth-grade girl. She apparently showed it to her friends, and they all had a good laugh at me. I was crushed, and I think that maybe that's where I decided that:

1. It's not safe to express my physical attraction to a girl.
2. I'm not worthy of a relationship.
3. It's wrong to like a girl.
4. I'm silly to think I can have a girlfriend.
5. Women betray me.
6. My love (and my toy ring) are not good enough.
7. I'm a failure.
8. My fantasies won't come true.
9. I can't have the woman I want. (For the next five or six years, my attempts to get girlfriends were about as successful.)

Sexual history .... I was told very matter of factly about the facts of life when I was four or five. From then on, I was more interested in making friends with girls than boys. When I reached adolescence, I fantasized about having a girl, but many years went by without one.

I didn't have a car, the courage, the money, the social graces, etc. Most of the girls I did get involved with would not have sex with me. One girl I cuddled with a lot for a few summers was my first intercourse partner. She was a Jehovah's Witness, about my age, and didn't want to have sex. I finally wasn't a virgin anymore, but I felt guilty for "making" her do something she didn't want to do. I doubt if I've really released the thought that it's bad for me to want and have sex.

Around twenty, I realized that all through my teens I had been unconsciously judging people (boys and girls). Some were better than me, and I was lucky if they acknowledged my existence. The other group wasn't as good as me, and although they would associate with me (since they were lucky that I acknowledged their existence), I didn't want to be seen too much with them because it would ruin my chances of moving up to a better standing. (In my own unconscious value world.)

Masturbation .... I didn't learn how to masturbate until I was sixteen or seventeen (much too late in my opinion), and like most kids, I decided I'd discovered something great. I was ashamed of it, because when my dad asked about the stains on my sheets, I denied it, and was very embarrassed. My best friend was the one who told me the details of how to masturbate. When I don't have a girlfriend, I masturbate about five times a week.

Church conditioning .... I didn't really have any "church conditioning" until after I'd done the LRT. At twenty-two, I didn't want monogamy, and I had a girlfriend who did. After a lot of counseling, one counselor suggested that we were "soul mates" (i.e. We always had been together throughout time, although we had perhaps lived some lifetimes apart). I latched on to this as a belief system, and spent the next two years trying to live by the data of the community of couples who believed that they were "like vibrations". I'm not sure exactly what they taught or believed, but here is how I mutated their instructions. This is what I thought I needed to do:

- Purge all thoughts of other women, and focus completely on my wife.
- Suppress or ignore my own desires, and turn over my life to God.
- Share all my possessions, or I'd just be alone and selfish.

And it got worse. I thought that:

- This community was the only path to God for me, so if I left it I'd be giving my life to satan, and I would never find my way back to God. Hence I was trapped somewhere I didn't want to be.
- All my resistance to the community and its data was a negative part of my mind that I had to ignore or fight. God wanted me to do things I didn't want to do, but should want to do.

I finally left this community to do what I felt like doing, (not being a husband or a father or monogamous, etc.). However I felt I was bad and a failure, a quitter. I felt not good enough and sinful. You name it, and I beat myself up with it.

More recently, I've judged myself as a wimp and a fool for getting involved with all that and selling out on myself. It's been a long road trying to recover from the guilt and self-hatred I generated and affirmed during that time.

8. BERT

Conception description .... Any thoughts I might have about my conception are pure speculation, since I haven't experienced any kind of recall of it. I do have a few speculations about "conception trauma", based on what I know about the circumstances. My mother was only seventeen, and my father nineteen. They were married, but my father was unemployed, so they were heavily dependent on my mother's parents for financial help during this period. My mother's parents looked down on my father, at least at first, since his family was poor and uneducated, while my mother's family were college-educated, professional people.

How my conception affects my sexuality .... I theorize that I was really a threat to my mother's already shaky security. That I got by "osmosis" from her the idea that I "shouldn't be", or that I "didn't belong there".

Birth description .... My mother tells me that my birth was easy, her labor lasting only five hours.

My Personal Lies are .... I AM NOT GOOD ENOUGH. I DON'T DESERVE TO BE LOVED. I AM TRAPPED AND I HAVE TO GET OUT OF HERE.

Feeding pattern .... I experienced a situation for a few months following birth which almost certainly evoked a third "Personal Lie". My mother breast-fed me, but unknown to her, her milk was defective and did not nourish me properly. The result of this was mild malnutrition and chronic digestive upset.

How my feeding pattern affects my sexuality .... I think I was convinced, very early on, that in the world outside the womb, "I can't get no satisfaction". Or even maybe, "When I try to get satisfaction, I get hurt".

Childhood incidents of sexuality .... The first sexual experience I can recall happened when I was five years old. There was a little girl named

Claudette who lived in the same apartment house that we lived in, and I often played with her. One day while we were playing, she said "Let's suck peters". What I thought she said was, "Let's soak peters." What this meant to me was, "Let's urinate on each other's penises." I didn't know at the time that she didn't have a penis.

This seemed like an interesting idea, so I said "yes". She took my hand and led me to a hiding place back behind the garage, where we both took our pants down and indeed urinated, but not on each other. I recall being disappointed at this discrepancy between what I thought she had proposed, and what we were doing. I don't recall noticing that she didn't have a penis. At any rate, when we had finished urinating, she got down on her knees in front of me and began to suck my penis. This was a somewhat shocking surprise to me. We didn't continue this for very long, and I don't recall getting any particular pleasure from it—I think I was far too flabbergasted.

Somehow I got the idea about what had happened that it wasn't really an OK activity. I think that by age five I had already absorbed the idea that my penis was somehow a "not-OK" part of my body. At any rate, I felt guilty about the experience, and confessed it to my mother, who seemed neither shocked nor indignant about it, but instead, rather sympathetic and reassuring toward me, and only mildly morally superior toward little Claudette. I think her attitude probably was, "You can't expect much better from these lower-class people around here, but let's not let Bert get all bent out of shape about it." At any rate, mother's reassurances were effective, and I didn't get all bent out of shape about it.

The only other sex-related childhood experience I can recall, happened when I was nine years old. The family who lived next door to my grandmother's house had a playhouse in their back yard, and I often played there with their children, Katherine and Jim. One day when Jim wasn't around, and Katherine and I were playing together in the playhouse, she suggested that we take off our clothes. We did. By this time, I was slightly acquainted with the genital differences between boys and girls, since it was my mother's custom, when she was out shopping, to take me into the restroom with her when she needed to urinate. So I had learned by then that female people didn't have penises. But I seem to recall being surprised to see that Katherine didn't have pubic hair—even though I had none myself.

Something else occured when I was nine years old which, though nonsexual, had a substantial influence on my sex life, as well as on other areas of my life. My grade in school took an achievement test, on the basis of which I and one of my classmates, whose name was Jay, were put up half a grade. We were told that in most parts of the test, our performance was of high-school level rather than fourth-grade level. So we left all our old classmates behind, and went into a class of strangers. I think Jay handled this sudden transition pretty well, but I didn't. I was very shy ("I'm not good enough. I don't deserve love."), and I found it very hard to make any new friends.

Thus began a period of very extreme social isolation which lasted throughout my teens—during the very period when my sexuality was developing very strongly. For most of my teens, Jay was literally my only friend. Along with this social isolation, however, occurred a period of precocious intellectual development. For example, I had special permission to take out books from the adult section of my hometown's public library, and I read just about everything I could get my hands on. I also had access to all the books.

Puberty . . . . By the time I was twelve I had bought and studied two of the best "marriage manuals" of the period: one by Hannah and Abraham Stone, whose title I don't remember, and the other, *Ideal Marriage* by Theodore Van de Velde. By the time I entered my teens, I had a pretty good, elementary knowledge of human sexual anatomy and physiology, including the mechanics of intercourse.

But as a result of the extreme reticence of these books to mention any but the most conventional sexual practices, I had no idea that there was such a thing as anal sex; that oral sex was a widespread practice considered perfectly normal by many people; that there was a name for the pleasant practice of playing with my genitals which I had discovered on my own; that a woman's breasts had anything to do with sexual activity (though they were fascinating to me, for reasons I didn't understand); that it was possible for a girl to get pleasure from playing with her genitals in a way analogous to the way I enjoyed playing with mine; or that it was enjoyable for a woman to have her genitals stimulated orally.

Another result of the "bookish" way I got my elementary sex education was, that the words that I first learned in the area of sexuality were the scientific terms, not the slang. I knew a lot about "having intercourse" for several years before I was sure that "fuck" meant the same thing. I knew what my "penis" was for several years before I knew I had a "cock", I knew what a "vulva" was for years before I knew what a "pussy" was. I knew what a "vagina" was for years before I ever heard of a "cunt". Even now, I habitually use the scientific terms unless I'm really turned on sexually.

My parents knew that I owned the two "marriage manuals". Consequently, neither of them ever gave me a lecture about "the birds and the bees," at least with regard to anatomy and physiology. My mother did give me a minilecture on sexual feelings when I was about thirteen years old, which I have always felt was very wise. It was pretty much as follows: "You're old enough now that you'll probably be starting to feel unfamiliar feelings toward girls.

This is perfectly normal. Don't worry about it." That was all the parental sexual instruction I ever got, except a much later injunction that I should never get anybody pregnant who I wasn't married to.

At this same period, I was reading novels whose authors just seemed to take it for granted that it was pretty much OK to have sex outside of marriage. I adopted this point of view myself, as a result of thinking about what I was reading. All this by about age thirteen. Although I had been masturbating (but not to orgasm), for maybe a couple of years, I didn't really "know what I was doing" until I was about thirteen. I had read in the Boy Scout Manual about two things which it called "self-abuse" and "nocturnal pollution", but I didn't connect either term with my own experience.

At about thirteen I had my first "wet dream". Soon after that, I ejaculated one evening when I was standing in front of the bathroom sink playing with myself. Immediately I realized that this was what the Manual had meant by "self-abuse", and I resolved never to do it again. However, it felt so good that I never made a serious attempt to live up to my resolution. But the negative attitude that I had absorbed stayed with me, so that until very recently (maybe the last couple of months), there was always some feeling of guilt and unworthiness associated in my mind with my masturbating.

Although at a purely intellectual level I had become fairly well-informed about sex (even perhaps a bit "sophisticated" in my opinions about sexual morality), at the level of real interaction with real girls, I was terrified and petrified. ("I'm not good enough, I'm not worthy of love or affection. If anyone appears to like me, it's a hoax, because I'm not worthy of it. If I ask for a date, the girl will just laugh at me, so I won't ask.")

On the one occasion during my teens when I did muster the courage to ask the girl I had "long worshipped from afar" for a date, she told me very sweetly and kindly that she already had plans for that occasion. I was devastated, and never tried for a date again during high school. What made all this even more painful for me was that all through high school, I had the worst case of acne that I have ever seen, before or since. I think maybe my body was "saying yes" to my conviction that I was completely unlovable.

First sexual experience .... After high school, I went to college for a year, by the end of which my parents had helped me all they could financially, and I decided to enlist in the army to save enough money to finish college. In December, 1948, I enlisted and signed up for training as a surgical technician. After this training, in the fall of 1949, I was assigned to Madigan Army Hospital at Fort Lewis, Washington. By this time, my acne was well on the way to clearing up, and I was feeling somewhat better about myself. I decided that my sex life had been all in my head for much too long, and that I was now going to lose my virginity.

I went on a weekend pass with a buddy up to Seattle, where without much difficulty we found a brothel. But when I got into the bedroom and onto the bed with the girl I was going to be with, I couldn't get an erection ("I'm not good enough, and I can't get no satisfaction."). The girl, a pretty black girl, asked me if this was the first time I had ever been with a woman, and I told her that it was. She told me not to worry, that it wasn't unusual for a man to be so apprehensive his first time that he couldn't get hard. She asked me of I'd like for her to "love me with her mouth". By this time I knew about oral sex—from my reading, of course—and I gratefully said "yes". So she gave me head. I told her how grateful I was, and my buddy and I left.

During the rest of my three and a half years in the army, the subsequent four years of college, and the next nine years, my sex life consisted of occasional visits to prostitutes, and masturbation. While I was in college, I dated quite a bit. Although I now had developed enough courage to ask women for dates, I hadn't yet developed enough courage to initiate a sexual relationship with any of the women I knew.

I never had any feeling of contempt or superiority toward any of the prostitutes whom I visited. But of course, there was also no emotional involvement with them. What was worst of all, the realization simply never occurred to me that the kind of sex that I was having with prostitutes, which was oriented purely toward my own pleasure, was not the kind of sex that would please any woman with whom I might have a real, loving relationship.

Sexual experiences . . . . My first real relationship with a woman developed about nine years after I came to work in California. I was thirty-six years old at the time, and although I wasn't sure how old June was, and didn't ask, I would guess that she was in her very late forties or very early fifties. She was divorced, sexually accomplished, and looking for a relationship which would be friendly, even affectionate to some degree, but centered on sex. I was sexually very unaccomplished, and still very much in the grip of my ancient beliefs that "I wasn't good enough," and "I didn't deserve love".

June accepted the role of my teacher—we both described her role very explicitly as that of my sexual teacher as well as my sexual partner. But since up to that time I had simply never learned how to hold off my orgasm in intercourse for even as long as one minute, her receiving pleasure from our sexual activity was very frustrating for her. Although I learned a lot from June about how to make love to a woman in foreplay, I was not able to learn during our relationship how to delay my orgasm long enough to be able to please her in intercourse.

The only things that kept our sexual relationship from being a complete disaster for both of us were that (1) I loved playing with her breasts and she loved being turned on that way, and (2) I loved giving her oral sex and she loved receiving it. But these activities were not sufficient; and as June became more and more frustrated with my prematurity, I became more and more frustrated with the role of the inept student of a more and more "antsy" teacher. My "gotta get out of here" response was very strongly evoked during the latter part of this relationship. So we had a very stormy, "off-again, on-again" time of it for our last couple of months. I still remember vividly her exasperated suggestion, delivered near the end of our relationship; "You'd really better find yourself some nice Jewish guy and get him to teach you how to fuck!" (She was Jewish).

It was during that "breakdown" period of the relationship with June that I met Jean. Within a month of meeting Jean, I had proposed marriage, and she had said "yes". Jean and I never "went all the way" before our wedding. In fact, all that we really did sexually was a lot of excited fondling and a lot of very beautiful, deep kissing. Although I was not romantically in love with Jean, I liked her a lot, and felt very comfortable with her, and the way she hugged and kissed me implied to me very strongly that when we got around to having sex, it could be wonderful.

The first time we had intercourse was on our wedding night. For Jean it was a disaster, since I got her very excited and then came almost immediately. During the nearly twenty years of our marriage before Jean became terminally ill, I gradually learned to delay my orgasm longer and longer, so that on many occasions I was able to last for ten to twenty minutes.

But the sad fact is that as I approached the goal of being able to satisfy her in intercourse, that goal receded. I think that during the entire twenty-year, sexually active period of our marriage, I succeeded in bringing Jean to climax in intercourse only four or five times. How I did bring her to orgasm was by masturbating her and by giving her oral sex. But even here we had problems; she simply would not tell or show me how she wanted me to stimulate her sexually, her belief being that it was "not her place" to tell me or show me, but rather my place, as a man, simply to "know". She also insisted that she couldn't even get anything out of masturbating herself, since, she said, masturbating only gave her very shallow orgasms which, far from satisfying her, only made her hunger for intercourse more ravenously.

She often said that she loved the way I gave her oral sex, and that whenever I felt like doing that, I should either let her know or just initiate it. But when I let her know that I wanted it, she more and more often "begged off", and when I simply started it, she more and more often asked to put it off until later. Maybe I was "doing it wrong". But I couldn't get her to talk with me about how I could "do it right". I recall when I made oral love to her for about forty-five minutes, and still wasn't able to bring her to orgasm. To be very honest, in the period just before Jean's cancer incapacitated her, sex with her had become for me almost a chore rather than a delight. And after that she was too sick for us to be able to make love.

Dovetailing Personal Lies with partner .... As far as our Personal Lies were concerned, we were perfectly matched for disaster. We each "knew", at gut level, that no one could really love us. Jean had been a battered child, from about age eight to sixteen, and had actually been sent by the court to live with an aunt and uncle for a while to get her away from her mother and stepfather—a fact perfectly designed to play hell with her self-esteem.

Jean's mother had left her real father when Jean was about three years old, so "men abandoned her". To get out of her intolerable home situation, she married Bill, a high school boyfriend, when she was not quite seventeen. He turned out to be abusive, terrified of having sex, and a "mama's boy", who spent much more time with his mother than with Jean. She had four children in just a little more than four years; two boys, two years apart, and then twin girls two years later. Before the twins were born—in fact probably before they were conceived—she left Bill.

There ensued for her then a sexually very active period, at the end of which she met and fell very deeply in love with a man named Paul. They lived together in a very beautiful, very close relationship for several months, during which she found that she was pregnant with the twins. But since she had been in a sexually very active period just before she met Paul, she wasn't at all sure that Paul was the father. She loved Paul so much that she felt she had to be honest with him about the fact that he might conceivably not be the twins' father. She told him this, and he couldn't handle it: he abruptly ended the relationship.

The shock of this was something that she didn't really get over for years, and perhaps to some degree not at all. For about two years after that she had no sex life at all, and tried to concentrate her mind and her emotions as completely as possible on spiritual growth. She later felt about this time in her life, that if she had not discovered "metaphysics", she would very probably have become suicidal. So Religious Science and it's approach to life helped her stay sane. But during this period she had four small children to take care of, and no marketable skills, and Bill was not paying the child support money that the court had awarded her at her divorce. She had to go on welfare.

Against her own beliefs and inclinations she became a "welfare cheat", since if she had been a "good citizen", and had tried to subsist on just the welfare payments without illegal employment in her home, she would have had to feed and clothe herself and four small children on about thirty dollars a month. (When I hear comfortably well-off people bitching about "welfare cheaters" and "people who'd rather collect welfare than work", my blood pressure starts climbing, although I know that there are some cheaters and lazy bums on welfare).

For a brief period of a couple of months she became a part-time prostitute, selling her body to men brought to her (and screened for her) by a couple of friends. She told me that all of the several men who became her clients were very kind and understanding towards her. After that, she became for seven years, the mistress and under-the-table business associate of Hank, a prosperous, married, business man. This was the period of her life about which she felt shame and regret—not because she was the mistress of someone whom she didn't love, but because she was "the other woman".

He began to insist that she behave almost as a prisoner in her own little house. For probably five years, her sub-exsistence completely depended on her being willing to do this. At the end of that time, she just couldn't take it any more, and told him so. They parted amicably—somehow during all the garbage they had become genuinely fond of each other. He gave her enough money to subsist on for a few months, but when that was gone, she had no means of support but the welfare payments which were totally inadequate for the needs of her little family. There ensued then a period of about two years, during which she and her four kids often did not know where their next meal was coming from. It was at the end of that two-year period that she and I met, pre-programmed for disaster.

As mentioned previously, we both came into our marriage convinced, way down deep, that we were unlovable. So we both tended to interpret whatever the other might do that hurt us, as coming out of dislike, hate, contempt, rather than out of the thoughtlessness or pain of the other. One of Jean's Personal Lies was "Men abandon me", and one of mine, which tends to be brought up very strongly in difficult relationships, is "I've got to get out of here, or I'll die". This was a combination sure to result in turmoil. One of the ways that my "I can't get no satisfaction" manifested itself was that whenever I came when I had intercourse with Jean, I felt sad and defeated because I hadn't brought her to orgasm.

One very serious problem area between us is I don't see quite how to relate to our "Personal Lies" as I understand them. This was that Jean was terrified of not being in control of whatever situation she was in, including our marriage. It would have been easy enough for me to mistake this for a simple, egotistical insistence on having her own way. But from the beginning, I realized that it probably came from the fact that her total life experience before we met had consisted of one catastrophe after another whenever she just let nature take its course. To make things worse, I had had an unusually long history of not having to account to anyone but myself; so a relationship in which a continual conflict over dominance was going on between us, was completely to be expected.

I am very highly susceptible to vulnerability in a woman. Not only is vulnerability a sexual turn on for me, but also it awakens very strongly in me feelings of tenderness and protectiveness. But showing her vulnerability was something that Jean couldn't allow herself to do; she couldn't show vulnerability and still be in control.

Only as her developing cancer left her more and more incapacitated did she seem able to relinquish control, and let me be simply tender and protective. Subsequently, as her illness got worse, we became closer and closer, and more and more able simply to love each other in an uncomplicated way. I want whatever new relationship I may enter, to be in this respect similar to the last few months of my marriage with Jean. I believe that this will be possible.

9. TOM

Conception description .... If I were a betting man, I would have to say it occurred when my parents felt they were doing what a husband and wife were supposed to do. I feel that my conception occurred without much feeling or desire to produce children. The sex was mechanical, and I was not planned.

How my conception affects my sexuality .... In the past, my sexuality was mostly mechanical. I was more concerned with technique than with emotions. Now I'm more concerned with emotions, and I let technique take care of itself.

Birth description .... I don't believe I was born when I wanted to be born, but rather when others wanted me to. I was not ready to be in this world.

How my birth affects my sexuality .... I was a late bloomer in regards to sex. I was twenty-three when I had my first intercourse with a woman. Up until then, I wasn't ready for sex. I felt inadequate. In fact, everything comes to me later in life than it does to most people.

My Personal Lie is .... I'M NOT WANTED OR GOOD ENOUGH.

How my Personal Lie affects my sexuality .... I withhold until I feel I am wanted, or good enough. I feel I have no sexual magnetism; that I am not good enough to have it. Therefore, I put the message out that I am no good at sex, and that you don't want me.

My biggest problem with sex is .... Foreplay. I want to immediately start to fondle and stroke the erogenous areas of my wife. She wants to be held and cuddled for a while before sexual stimulation. I also have a big problem with the lack of spontaneity or lust in our relationship.

Earliest memories of sex .... My earliest recollection of sex was when I was in the fifth grade, nine or ten years old. I was climbing a pole to get something at the top. I think it was a tetherball pole, and I was going to untangle it at the top. Climbing up, I remember getting a strange sensation in my groin, and not knowing what it was. It felt good. The sensation increased when I slid down the pole.

Church conditioning .... It was a sin if you had sex out of wedlock and for pleasure. Sex was only for procreation purposes and anything else was taboo. Thinking about sex and sexual attraction was also a sin, and I would go to hell if I did any of the above.

Parental conditioning .... My mother and grandmother did not prepare me for sex at all. Sex to them was as the church said. I educated myself by listening to what older kids said, and by reading pornographic literature.

Embarrassing situations with sex .... I can't say I have had any one most embarrassing experience with sex. My sex life has a whole section that is comic.

I was into my sexual revolution. We read literature and saw movies showing sexual positions and techniques. We tried whip cream, chocolate, strawberry, grapes, the missionary position, from behind, standing, and sitting positions to total disaster. All we could do was laugh at ourselves or get angry. I got angry at times because I felt I failed to satisfy her.

If I had to pick a particular incident, it would have to be the time we were having sex with me behind her. I was to withdraw from her before my climax, and ejaculate on her back like we saw in a movie. Well, I withdrew from her the instant before I climaxed and ejaculated all over the wall across the room. I missed her completely. I just wanted to die. Now we had a bigger mess to clean up, and it left stains on the wall. I think they are still there. This occurred early in my relationship with my wife.

10. JAMES

Conception description . . . . I was unwanted by my father at conception. This has caused me to feel distant from my parents. I also have the thought that my father was not loving towards my mother when it came to sex. My thought is that his sex was mainly for his pleasure, without concern for my mother's feelings.

How my conception affects my sexuality . . . . I have had sex and intimacy confused most of my life.

Birth description . . . . I was a RH factor baby, and although they did not give me a transfusion, I know that I was in opposition to my mother in the womb, and separated at birth. They thought I might need a transfusion, and kept me in the hospital for nine days.

How my birth affects my sexuality . . . . I had the thought that I hurt women. I felt like I could never get enough sex. It was as if sex was my source of nourishment, or perhaps it was the transfusion I thought I needed and never got. For me to feel that a woman accepted me, I needed to know that she was willing to have sex with me. It didn't matter if we actually did it or not, as long as I knew she was willing.

My Personal Lie is . . . . I HURT WOMEN.

How my personal Lie affects my sexuality is . . . . I could have a very loving and satisfying sexual relationship with a woman, and she could feel very much in love with me, only to have me leave. It seems as if my desire is to have a woman fall in love with me at whatever cost, so that I can leave and hurt her.

My biggest problem with sex and my Personal Lie . . . . Sex leaves me feeling unsatisfied and incomplete. The intimacy and nourishment I would expect from the sex isn't there and I feel cheated. This causes me to continue my search for the nourishment in yet another woman, hurting the woman I am with.

My Sexual Eternal Law is . . . . MY ALIVENESS AND MY SEXUALITY IS A PLEASURE FOR ME AND FOR THE WOMAN I LOVE.

11. EVELYN

Conception description . . . . My father wanted sex when my mother didn't. Then, when she was pregnant, he didn't want to have sex. So maybe I believe that since when I came into existence my father quit wanting sex with my mom, there must be something about me that made my father non-sexual.

How my conception affects my sexuality . . . . I have an image of my conception as being a flash of white light, followed with a feeling of pure divine energy and inspiration—power. This is my sexuality, my life force. My father turned away from it—it was un-sexual to him. So maybe my thought is that my sexual energy and aliveness turns men off, which it often does. I feel rejected in my sexual relationships. When I feel sexual, my partner doesn't.

Birth description . . . . In some of my initial rebirths, I had the vague feeling that I had been sexually abused when I was a child, but I couldn't remember anything. Recently, in a rebirth, I had a memory of feeling beat up by my obstetrician and nurses when I was born. I felt assaulted for being alive. I realized then that this was the connection I had with childhood sexual abuse. I felt sexually abused at birth. My life energy and spirit were ignored, and I was treated like a hunk of meat with no life. Also, at birth I was separated from my mother.

How my birth affects my sexuality . . . . I have put this on men in some of my sexual relationships. Men don't treat me as a person—just a body with no spirit. And when men haven't treated me as just a body, I still fear that all they care about is their own pleasure, and not my spirit. So in sex I feel very fearful that I will be beat up. As a result, my vagina won't relax, and intercourse is painful. I get hurt when I have intercourse.

I create separation in my relationships. I am always longing for a better connection—something more—I feel so separate from my husband. We are so separate, we hardly can get together for sex. I have the thought that men hurt me, so it is terrifying for me to have sex.

Sex almost always feels like a struggle to me. I feel numb a lot when I am touched, and I feel like I want to go to sleep. Perhaps this is related to anesthesia. Also, the feelings I had about my birth are that I was held back and I couldn't get out—I always feel like I have to work to enjoy sex—it takes so much effort to get to sex. I feel clamped off, and I can't breathe when I'm having sex. Sex is a struggle and is not much fun—exactly my thoughts about birth. Yuck, I hate it.

My Personal Lie is .... I'M NOT GOOD ENOUGH.

How my Personal Lie affects my sexuality .... I never feel good enough. In sex, I don't feel womanly enough or passionate enough or sexy enough or loving enough or caring enough or enough of a lover. I don't do enough. I always feel inadequate, and then my husband is never good enough, never does enough, never loves me enough. He just isn't enough no matter what he does. Basically, I'm not good enough to have a wonderful sexual relationship, and since he loves me, he obviously isn't good enough either.

My biggest problem with sex is .... Being afraid of it and all the junk it brings up. Sex is a miserable affair for both of us. The way this fits my Personal Lie is, I'm not good enough to have pleasurable sex in my relationship.

My Sexual Eternal Laws are .... I AM GOOD ENOUGH TO HAVE A WONDERFUL, SEXUAL RELATIONSHIP. SINCE I AM GOOD ENOUGH, I CAN ALWAYS MOVE THROUGH MY BLOCKS TO SEXUAL PLEASURE. I AM GOOD ENOUGH TO HAVE SEXUAL PLEASURE.

12. DANIEL

Conception description .... My father was feeling that there was not enough time to complete his life. He was about to go into the hospital for the third time with tuberculosis.

How my conception affects my sexuality .... I feel like I am his extension of the thought, "I'm not going to make it". Basically, the way my father attempted to insure his immortality was through me.

All my issues about sex and intercourse center around time. I feel I won't last long enough to make my partner happy or satisfy her. My sex case is an extension of "I'm not going to make it".

Birth description .... My birth was accomplished very quickly, without an obstetrician. Forty-five minutes exactly, from the time the waters broke until I was born. I was premature and small—under five pounds. I was born at 6:15 in the morning.

How my birth affects my sexuality .... Most of my sexual experiences have been high intensity for up to one hour maximum. After an hour's time,

I usually experience a loss of sexual appetite for a while. Also, my frequency of sex seems to go in binges, changing from every day for three or four days, to nothing for a week to ten days. My experience with extended foreplay generally leads to some sensation of pain, since my first touching experience with the nurses was a little like sandpaper.

As I stated earlier, my biggest problem with sex has always been the time issue. I feel that there is not enough time, or I have a sense of urgency, or I think it is the wrong time or the wrong place. This corresponds perfectly with my birth, since I was almost born in the cab.

Since my birth was so fast, I had the sense that most things, particularly sex, were an outcome rather than an experience. Therefore, I was extremely attached to the orgasm, and not what was building up to the orgasm. For a long time I had no use for foreplay, and actually despised too much touching. Most of my sexual experiences prior to rebirthing lasted thirty minutes or less. For many years I prefered masturbation to sex with a partner.

My anxiety over being smothered used to prevent me from enjoying several positions. Since I was not allowed to bond with my mother, and never received her breast, I actually had an aversion to large-breasted women, and would generally refuse to fondle or touch them in any way during sex. My thought about not getting what I want played out in my sex life. My partners and I were never on schedule. Also, I always have believed women aren't ready when I am.

My Personal Lie is .... I AM A DISAPPOINTMENT.

How my Personal Lie affects my sexuality .... All the above would prove that I am a disappointment sexually.

My Sexual Eternal Law is .... I AM A WONDERFUL SURPRISE AS A LOVER.

13. ARNETTE

Conception description .... I was conceived in my aunt's apartment. My parents were not married. They were under the influence of alcohol. They were both musicians. I'm pretty sure my mother was in love with someone other than my father. It was a social disgrace to be pregnant and not married.

How my conception affects my sexuality .... I have duplicated my conception by marrying someone while I was in love with another man. I fall in love with musicians at sight. Music and alcohol have an aphrodisiac effect on me. I am attracted to socially unacceptable situations for sex. Most significant is my belief that I shouldn't exist. I do not express the "real" me. I do not want others to see me. Therefore I attract men who don't know the real me, and then I'm disappointed.

Birth description .... My birth was normal, natural and easy, but not without some pain for my mother. My father was ten feet away and could hear everything, but not see it. They were expecting a boy. I was born at 5:40 PM, shortly before dinner time. He heard the doctor tell my mother to "push" several times. I did not have a name because they only had a boy's name picked out The nurses pressured my mother to come up with a girl's name. All she could think of was Punch and Judy. So she told them Judy (Judith). Later, I hated the name, and changed it to Arnette. Mother did not nurse me—she had no milk, and I was allergic to my formula.

How my birth affects my sexuality .... The way these events have been duplicated in my life are many. I assumed a male identity. I do not remember people's names when I first meet them. I sense my world through my ears mostly. I find sex normal, natural and easy. I was not satisfied sexually for much of my second marriage.

My Personal Lies are .... THERE IS SOMETHING WRONG WITH ME and I'M NOT GOOD ENOUGH.

HOW MY PERSONAL LIE AFFECTS MY SEXUALITY .... I liked sex and thought it was natural. I figured there must be something wrong with me because my parents, church, and society were not in agreement. Men wanted me for all the wrong reasons. I felt I had to look like a beauty queen. I did not feel good enough just the way I was. I always chose partners who had something wrong with them, which kept us apart. When I get a lot of attention from men (proving that I'm good enough), I create something wrong with me.

Father's attitudes toward sex .... He likes it so much he says if he didn't get it, he'd rather be dead. He would placate my mother so she wouldn't withhold sex from him. While I was growing up, it was not acceptable for me to enjoy sex. "If a man looks at you, he's thinking about taking you to bed."

Mother's attitudes toward sex .... "All men want is sex." She doesn't like men or sex. When she was angry, she would withhold sex.

Paternal grandmother .... Frigid and proud of it! Church and society say that sex outside of marriage is wrong!

Parental conditioning .... The way my parents' attitudes effected me was that I found that all men (except my present husband) wanted to have sex with me, and sex was the most important aspect of our relationship. I felt used and very sad.

Oedipal period .... Between four and six years old, my father caught me masturbating and he was very angry. I was interested in sex play with other children, but knew it was wrong, so I did it in hiding and felt guilty.

Between seven and ten years old .... Because of my strict Catholic training about sex (a mortal sin in thought, word or deed), I became increasingly guilt-ridden about all sexual experiences. However, this was not enough to stop the behavior.

I had sex play and investigation with other girls, or by myself. If a boy approached me, or even discussed the subject, I would feel fear, disgust, shame and repulsion. At one point, I was very interested in sex play. So much so, that I left home one morning at dawn to meet a girlfriend for this purpose. If I remember correctly, there was a lot of sex play going on within her family (between brothers and sisters). This fascinated me.

Puberty .... At eleven years old, I made the transition to boys. I had a lot of difficulty with ambivalence—feeling desire and repulsion at the same time. I was turned on but felt disgusted. I was in seventh grade, and the nuns were bearing down hard on anything to do with the body. Very strict behavior and dress codes. I was fascinated by all the naughty girls in my class, but I did not want to behave like them. I had a terrifying experience that year in a neighborhood park. A male classmate (who resembled my pediatrician) tried to molest me. I was very well-developed and was wearing a sweater. It had a profound effect on me. I hid my breasts from then on. I felt rage, guilt and disgust toward the boy.

From twelve to fifteen years .... boys, boys, boys. I couldn't get enough. I loved making out. I had lots of guilt if it went beyond kissing. This had no effect on my behavior, though. Any indication of my sexuality made my mother very upset. She would look at me with intense disgust. She had a lot of anger about it, too.

I was always in trouble with my parents because I would disobey them in order to be with my boyfriends. I was grounded and punished so much I decided to get even by going "on strike" and not seeing my friends. My father was the one to give punishment during this period, and he call me a "slut" at one point. I was still a virgin. At fifteen, I "fell in love" with my uncle and he with me. We had no sex. One kiss only, which shocked us both.

Sexual history .... At sixteen and seventeen, I had a very intense sexual affair with my uncle. I wanted intercourse, but he felt it was improper. We broke up, and they adopted a child. My aunt was my fantasy mother.

At eighteen, I dated lots of men of all ages. I had no intercourse and found dating boring. I was still in love with my uncle.

At nineteen, I married someone I had known only a short time. I felt we would be good business partners (and we were). He raped me on our wedding night. I was a virgin up until then.

Between twenty and twenty-seven, I was married to him. I pretended to enjoy sex with him. I hated most of it because he was into strange things like porno books, films, props and picture-taking. I felt degraded. I objected verbally. I always had a vaginal orgasm, after the birth of my first child, when we had sex.

At twenty-eight, I divorced my first husband and was re-united with my uncle.

Between twenty-nine and thirty-three, I married my uncle. Sex with him was wonderful at first. Our life became very strained and our sex life deteriorated after a few years because of impotence and premature ejaculation. I would often create something wrong with my husband's behavior in order to be angry, and then I would not want to have sex.

From thirty-four to the present, I have been separated. One of his daughters comes between us emotionally. We are still in a primary relationship with little or no sex.

14. THERESA

Conception description .... My parents were really young when they went out. They were not married when I was conceived. My mother was seventeen and my father was twenty-four. Grandpa didn't want them to get married, because he didn't want his daughter to marry a Catholic. When they got pregnant, they got married. My father was from a lower class than my mom. They were in love when they conceived me. I never felt unwanted. My mom was frightened, but she wanted to have sex with her first boyfriend before she got married.

My father felt trapped and later he struggled to stay. He would drink, and he and mom would fight. He then would feel guilty and bad because they had to get married. I feel responsible that my parents didn't get along, and had to get married because of me. My mother never got to be a nurse like she wanted to.

How my conception affects my sexuality .... My relationships get sexual very quickly. It is a rush to get committed. I am bi-sexual. I have been with women since I was nineteen. I fall in love with both girls and boys.

Birth description .... I was three weeks late. It was a pretty straightforward birth, except my mom had to be snipped. She hemorrhaged and couldn't deliver the placenta. The doctor drugged her and pulled it out. My thought is, men hurt women, and I get blamed. The doctor hurt my mom, but I got blamed.

How my birth affects my sexuality .... I get committed very fast. Then I feel trapped and suffocated. I feel that my father felt that way. I always am looking for a way out. I pick partners who are monogamous. Then they get hurt when I flirt and go with other women. I need playtime so I don't feel suffocated. I got hurt in my first homosexual relationship when my partner played around. Because I was late, I will stay in relationships longer than I think I should. When I come out, I play around, and then I hurt my partner like I hurt my mom.

My Personal Lie is .... I AM BAD AND NO GOOD.

How my Personal Lie affects my sexuality .... I get to be bad if I play around or have affairs. I get to hurt my partner. I get to be bad if I get committed, because then I can't stick to it, and I leave.

My biggest problem with sex and my Personal Lie .... I can be bad if I withhold sex, or don't want it, or I don't want to do it because they expect it.

Oedipal Period .... When we were four and five, we would play horses and rub our genitals together. My brother and I would crawl in bed together and tickle each other when we were five and six. We took baths together. After awhile, Dad separated us. The first time I noticed the difference between a boy and a girl was when I was four, and a boy who was circumcised showed me his "dinger".

First sexual experience .... When I was sixteen, I had sex with my boyfriend who I had gone out with since I was thirteen. My dad was real jealous.

My boyfriend was two years older. It was a struggle because he was a good Catholic boy. He wanted to get married before he had sex. I talked him into sex.

Masturbation . . . . I started experimenting when I was lying in bed at eleven or twelve.

Parental conditioning . . . . Dad was brought up Catholic, and he had guilt and embarrassment about sex. He couldn't talk to us about it. My mother was Methodist, and she was very embarrassed to talk about sex, and even about menstruation. I didn't get my first period until I was sixteen. I got my second period at seventeen.

Most embarrassing sexual situation . . . . I was with a married woman and her husband came in.

15. CHRIS

Conception description . . . . My father wasn't around a lot—he was in his early twenties and loved to party. This meant going out drinking and flirting. He was having several affairs, so my mother was fairly shut down—she was feeling isolated and alone.

The night I was conceived, my father was high on alcohol, and my mother was shut down and hurt.

How my conception affects my sexuality . . . . I had the thought that the men in my life must be high in order to enjoy sex with me. "Getting high" together seemed the normal thing to do in order to enjoy the sexual experience fully.

The sexual experience never seemed quite "real". I wasn't in touch with my true, natural feelings. I was more addicted to the feeling of being "swept away".

In the past, I've attracted men who weren't around a lot. They were usually seeing other women, which made me feel inadequate and isolated. I seemed to be always waiting for them to either show up or call.

Birth description . . . . My father was living two lives—on with my mother and one with another woman, both pregnant. He was into guilt and denial at this point. He was denying that I was his child. Mom had made the decision to divorce him. She was nineteen, with one baby and another on the way.

She felt as if her whole world was shattered, and was waiting for me to be born before she finally took action.

She was into denial also, not wanting to face what was going on. She felt totally helpless and full of grief. I was six weeks late. I felt as if I had to hold back until she was in a different state of mind. I had planned to make the moment as joyful as possible—I always have been one to pick the most opportune moment, being the "ham" that I am!

I felt "wanted" by Mom, but Dad didn't want anything to do with me. I felt that Dad would have stuck around if I had been a boy. Even at my birth, I never really liked my dad. I guess I was picking up on all of the hurt Mom felt.

The doctor gave Mom sodium pentothal, and I was induced. Even being induced, I was still being stubborn about coming out. It took an additional six hours for me to come out. Like I said earlier, timing was important. The moment I did come out, everyone in the room was laughing. The doctor had the thought, "Well, this is a first!" This thought has affected me in many ways. I have always managed to be a "first" in my relationships. (First "white" girl, first American girl, first affair, etc..)

How my birth affects my sexuality . . . . The ways my birth experience has affected my relationships became real clear when I re-created my parents' situation a couple of years ago. I met a married man, fell in love, and became pregnant. He felt as though he was living two lives. He came very close to leaving his wife to be with me. I just had to understand subconsciously how my own father and his lover had felt—I HAD to make them "right."

I feel very closed-in when a relationship is six weeks old. I get confused and depressed. Once I pass this stage however, the situation gets lighter, and the relationship starts "moving."

I've left almost all of my relationships—the way my father left me. I've been in almost total denial most of my life—never trusting my "gut," and never seeing any relationship as it was. I felt my parents' relationship was based on lust, and most of my past relationships were also.

My Personal Lie is . . . . I'M NOT GOOD ENOUGH AS A WOMAN.

The effect of my Personal Lie on my sexuality . . . . This underlying thought has affected my relationships in many ways. In my younger years, I was very rebellious in my relationships. I always went for the "underdog"—always picking someone who wasn't good enough because I thought I wasn't good enough.

I was very, very insecure with men. My whole self-esteem was based on whether the man wanted me sexually, I decided I would be the "best" lover out there, because I felt that sex was all I had to offer.

I created one relationship that was totally abusive—physically, mentally and emotionally—because I thought I was worthless. I created another relationship where I was put on a pedestal—adored. I spent the first year building the pedestal, and the last two years trying to tear myself off of it. One extreme to the other, knowing all the time that I wasn't good enough to maintain the facade.

Church conditioning . . . . I was brought up as a Catholic and came from a very religious family. Sex was a big secret, never talked about. As a young child, I could "smell" it if anything sexual was going on.

I was playing out my mother's unconscious sexual guilt. If she had a man over, I was always sneaking around the corner—watching and listening. I never missed a thing! I was constantly walking in on my mother when she was with a man. Her reaction gave me the message that she was doing something wrong, and I was getting in trouble for witnessing her "sin." The connection that I made was that love and anger go together. Sex causes people to get angry.

In my own relationships, my partner and I would never talk about sex. Sex was something that just happened—it was "wrong" to talk about it. In the past, I would create my partner either being angry with me before sex or afterwards, because somehow this would make it "OK."

My first sexual relationship . . . . The summer after high school graduation—I was seventeen. My best friend at that time was sexually active, and my curiosity was growing about this thing called sex.

I had been going to this club—Los Gringos—where most of the Latins hung out. I was practicing flirting and learning how to move my body in sensuous ways to the Latin music. I met an older American named Dick at the club. He was very good-looking, and I made the decision to have sex with him the moment I met him.

He had lost his wife in a car accident recently, and was full of guilt because he had been the one driving. He was busy drinking himself into further denial. Sometimes when he was really drunk, he would call me by his wife's name.

I found myself fantasizing about him and the relationship—wanting to turn the lustful-type thoughts into love thoughts. I wasn't seeing the relationship the way it really was at all.

The night we had sex we were both drunk. He more so than me. We had just left a bar and were in the car making out, only this time he was more persistent. I was just letting it happen, pretending I didn't know what I was doing.

He was very rough, and manipulated me on top of him with the steering wheel in my back. I just kind of sat on his penis, he reached orgasm, and that was that! I felt totally disappointed and told him so. I remember being real quiet, and him asking me how I felt. I kept saying "That's all there is to it? It hurts. It doesn't feel good at all." This made him very angry, and he drove me home. The whole experience left me confused and disappointed.

My most embarrassing sexual situation .... My sister was house-sitting for friends of my parents for a couple of months, and I was still seeing Dick once in a while. One day, we went to my parents' friends house to have sex.

Dick had left, and I was on my way out when I ran into my mother and sister right outside the door. I was so embarrassed and full of guilt that I had been "busted". My mother sensed immediately that I had done something wrong, and started questioning me. "Why was I there, and who had I been with?" I told her everything except that we had had sex, but I felt that she knew.

Even to this day, I'm always scared that she's going to "walk in on me" when I have someone over.

16. NANCY

Conception description .... My father being furious that my mother was pregnant again, I sensed his fear and unhappiness, and my mother's partial withdrawal from me so as not to make him more unhappy. (She was secretly pleased.)

Decisions:

1. I'm a mistake.
2. My existence makes others angry and unhappy.
3. I'm not wanted.
4. I don't want to be here.
5. This is all my fault. To correct it and win my father, I must be perfect.

How my conception affects my sexuality . . . .

1. I was never with the right man.
2. My partner was almost always angry at me, so I denied myself to please him.
3. I created almost being sexually abused at age four by a man who won my trust.
4. The men I loved always left me. Many times I had the feeling that I didn't want to be there, but I didn't act on the feelings.
5. Anything that went wrong, I was to blame.
6. I didn't believe I deserved to have what I really wanted.

Birth description . . . . I was the third baby. My birth was a normal, head-down one, with an easy labor. My mother had anethesia only at the last moment. I came quickly and easily. Momentarily, they told my mother not to push so the doctor could get there on time. This hurt and infuriated me, and I strongly felt that my delivery team "were stupid!" I distinctly wanted to slug the obstetrician in the face. He said I had a cute nose and I've always hated my nose. My back was hurt prenatally, and again when I was held back at birth. My father was waiting in the waiting room, and was very happy to have a girl. He cried when he first saw me, but I had already decided he was not to be trusted. My love for him has been suppressed since before birth. I roomed in with my mother, who unsuccessfully tried to nurse me. She gave up at one week and gave me a bottle. This was very traumatic.

Decisions:

1. Everybody is stupid.
2. I can do it myself, why won't you let me?
3. My mother can't give me what I really want and need even though she loves me.
4. I can't do things the way I want or have what I want.
5. Nobody cares about me.
6. I'm angry like my dad.
7. I have to deny myself like my mom.

Oedipal period . . . . When I was four years old, a real estate agent who was holding open houses for us won my trust, lured me into the garage, and was about to molest me when a neighbor stopped him. I was very frightened, and my father acted like nothing happened. I felt guilty, and was terrified for a long time that the man would come back and hurt me. No one dealt with my feelings. It was as though nothing had happened, so I decided I was bad and if I trusted someone, they would hurt and abuse me.

Puberty .... In junior high and high school, I was a good girl and a straight "A" student. When I dated, I only kissed and necked, feeling very guilty even though I enjoyed it. My parents taught me nothing about sex, and it was never discussed in our home. I got my period at age ten while my mother was away on a trip, so I hid in my room for five days. Nobody seemed to notice that I was hiding.

My father told me when I was in high school that boys only wanted one thing. He did nothing but make me feel disapproved of for growing up. I was terrified I'd get pregnant doing absolutely nothing, until I realized one day that that wasn't possible. When I was pregnant three years ago, I was embarrassed around my father because then he knew for sure I'd had sex! He taught me to suppress my female energy, because it was just going to get me in trouble.

Sexual history .... My first experience with intercourse was the best sexual experience I've ever had. It was when I was twenty, with my high school sweetheart, by a stream in the mountains. We always had great sex. He left me while I was in college and we were engaged. I never saw him again.

My next relationship was with an older man. The sex was great for a few months. Then, even though I was interested, he never really was again. He left me after three years. I had another three-year relationship which was extremely passionate, and occasionally almost abusive, with a man who was married and separated. He was cheating on me two or three times a week with strangers, despite the fact that we often had sex two times a day. At the end of three years and one miscarriage, he confessed his infidelity. I was crushed, and moved away to Hawaii to get over him. I didn't date again for four years.

The next relationship was my marriage. He never really separated from his family and made a commitment to me. He constantly criticized me, and could never get his job and money act together. Sex was passionate until our daughter was born, then it was virtually non-existent. Serious problems with my pregnancy and daughter, plus my fear of loss, plus all the other problems already mentioned, broke up the marriage. He left me eight months ago. Since then he has escalated his emotional abuse, and been neglectful of Ashley. Presently, I have no sexual relationship, just several men who are good friends.

17. MARYBETH

Conception description . . . . My mother's Personal Lie is a combination of I'm not good enough/I'm guilty/I can't do it right. She was raised Catholic, and seriously entertained the idea of being a nun. She grew up the second of seven children, on the wrong side of the tracks in upstate New York. She was sexually abused by her brothers as a child. Her father was distant, and she wanted her brothers to love her. Instead, the instigator brother hated her, from his own guilt and fear, I guess. She was very pretty and had a voluptuous figure, which made her very self-conscious. She was shy, but was thought to be stuck up when she was in high school.

She met my dad while she was working at the theater. He wanted to talk to her and take her home, but she ignored him. He kept coming back. My dad always has liked a challenge. He buttered up her friends till they convinced her to be nice to him. He was born in Augusta, Georgia, and raised in rural farm country.

My father was raised as an only child. He was active, outgoing, friendly, good-looking and popular in school. He had joined the Air Force, and was stationed in New York when he met my mother. I don't know what my father's Personal Lie would be, but it has something to do with being safe to love and be close to people. He is friendly to all, but not close to any.

My parents married in May, and I was born March 22, three weeks late. My mother was almost nineteen when she married, and my dad was twenty-one. I was conceived within the first few weeks of their marriage. My mother was of a mixed mind about sex—I think she was anticipating something wonderful, but was scared due to her inexperience, her childhood abuse, and her Catholic upbringing.

Unfortunately for her, my father's previous experience had not made him a warm, tender, sensitive lover. He knew what he wanted, and didn't take much time to set the stage or prepare my mother. I think she expected or hoped for something more romantic and loving. This insensitivity must have brought back all her feelings of anger, confusion, sadness, and longing for love associated with her earlier abuse. I think she feels she doesn't deserve to be loved.

How my conception affects my sexuality is . . . . My first experience of sex was very similar to the above. Mike and I met when I was fifteen, almost sixteen. He was seventeen. We dated for one year, and planned to marry when I graduated from high school. We had necked heavily and done everything, we thought, except have intercourse. We were both virgins and very naive. I held off, wanting to wait for marriage. It finally got down to—if you won't, I know somebody who will. A girl we worked with was more than willing. I was very confused. It was very important to me to be his first love and last love, but I felt pushed into something I wasn't ready for. I gave in.

We borrowed someone's apartment. I didn't feel right about using their bed, so we lay on the floor. I was scared and nervous, and so was he. I wanted moonlight, roses, candles and romance—I got quick and painful. I felt so horrible—I think I wanted to die. Instead, I got slightly drunk and cried. He felt like the heel he was, and offered to take me out of state and marry me that night. Sex for me became associated with pain, both physical and emotional. Not to mention the GUILT! I had attended six years of Catholic school, and all I had heard about sex was how bad it was. I had also thought about being a nun, and even a saint. Had I blown it!

I think a lot of the foundations for my walls were laid at that time against men and intimacy. I felt very alone, and didn't know who I could talk to about all the things I was feeling. Fortune and fate both smiled on me the third time we had sex. My parents were out of town for Easter, and I had the house to myself.

Our second time was in the back seat of a car, so the third time was the first time I felt comfortable with the setting and could relax some. We took more time. He was also more relaxed, and it was romantic. I felt loved and beautiful and wanted. And very vulnerable.

Fate stepped in when I conceived that night. I'm barely seventeen, I have sex three times, I'm a high school junior, I'm Catholic, and I'm pregnant and unmarried. And very scared and full of guilt. I don't remember being angry about it—I felt that it was God's punishment of me for sinning, and that I deserved to be punished. Maybe some of the thoughts I'm now having about "It's not safe to love and be loved" were being played out then.

I loved Mike and he loved me. I got pregnant, and he had to go to work full time and marry me and quit college. We both got hurt by love, so to speak. It took me years to get over a lot of my negative feelings about sex.

The older I got, the more anger toward men started surfacing. I figured it was because I felt that men had "used" me for sex, and I was angry at them, and at myself for allowing it. The major way my conception affected my sexuality is my anger at men. I have turned that anger on myself for most of my life. Anger has not been an emotion I've known how to deal with. Since my original source of anger appears to be my father, I've been stuffing it since birth.

My father and I have always maintained a distant, friendly relationship. As the oldest of eight, I was the one he depended on to help out, to take care of things and be responsible for everyone. I have some anger about being thrust into that role at such an early age. My father always called me Sis—almost like I was the sister he never had.

I think that anger is always very close to the surface in my relationships with men. Anger and fear of being hurt or used or rejected. For years I associated love with pain. I even heard myself make a statement once, about two years ago, that shocked even me. Someone asked me if I loved the man I was dating, and I said, "I don't know. It doesn't hurt, and the way I know how much I loved someone is by how much it hurts!"

That was about the time I came across Master Minding. I did a lot of work on what love looked like to me, and what I wanted it to look like. I started doing image work. And writing—pages and pages—trying to release a lot of junk from my mind and body. That May, I did my first LRT. And the process has continued—layer after layer. I realized recently, during my fifth LRT, that I had always associated a queasy feeling in the pit of my stomach with being in love. I know now that it is really anxiety and fear.

In spite of all this, I have had some fun, light, and sexually enjoyable relationships with men. Usually lasting under three months. I think, in general, that it is easiest for me to have sex in relationships that are not intimate. I relax more when there is distance—either emotional or physical—in the sense of not being able to see much of each other. I did have several very intense relationships. What I tended to do was lose myself, my identity, trying to be who I thought my partner wanted me to be, instead of relaxing and being who I was.

I have a lot of clearing to do about men, sex, anger, relationships, the past, my parents, my kids, etc. I will take another chance, I always do, but not before I integrate the thought that change is safe. Then I'll know it's safe to change my past ways of relating, and do things in a NEW, SAFE, SPECTACULARLY FUN, EASY WONDEROUS WAY.

18. LINDA

Conception description . . . . This is just speculation, as I don't know how my mom felt about sex. My feeling is that she either didn't enjoy it, or didn't feel OK about enjoying it. Probably she knew she might be fertile when I was conceived, but either wanted the closeness to my father after being gone all summer, or felt she didn't want sex, but "couldn't" say no—and I was conceived.

What I've been told about my conception is that Mom had been at her mom's in Wisconsin with my older sister for the summer, and Dad was working in Alaska. She had gotten home, left my sister with a friend, and she and Dad had taken a train trip to Fairbanks, just for one night. The hotels were full because the fair was on, and they could only find a room with single beds. Mom said they shared a single bed, and that's how I was conceived.

She also says the hotel owner thought they were on their honeymoon, so they must have been happy to be together.

How my conception affects my sexuality . . . . I find I have mixed feelings about sex—a push/pull feeling. I want it, but it's not worth the risk of getting pregnant. And the responsibility for not getting pregnant seems to end up on me, rather than eagerly and positively being shared by my mate. We have come to no good solution.

Birth description . . . . I felt my dad wanted a boy—he already had a daughter, and I was number two.

How my birth affects my sexuality . . . . I never tried to be feminine, and felt weird when I did try. Like dirty or revolting inside. I'd help dad—fix cars, dig holes etc. I was more his helper than either of my two younger brothers.

My Personal Lie is . . . . I'M A DISAPPOINTMENT AS A WOMAN.

How my Personal Lie affects my sexuality . . . . I don't act or dress sexy, and feel self-conscious if I do. I don't climax easily. I feel like I'm not everything that the man I'm with would want in a woman. Even though men tell me it feels real good to make love to me, I feel like something is missing. I felt this way a lot more in the past than I do now.

My biggest problem with sex . . . . I have mixed feelings about sex. It brings up "stuff", so I tend to avoid it, and I don't feel good about that. I feel guilty about doing it just for fun; without feeling loving or just because he or I might be horny. This turns me off mentally. It feels revolting, immoral and not right.

I have a resistance to sex because, in the past, it has been frustrating, and I remember that subconsciously, and don't want to go through it again. Also, it's always a question of "Am I fertile?" What a pain. I'm using the ovulation method with a diaphragm backup. I don't like leaving the diaphragm in for eight hours, as it constipates me. It's a hassle to get the diaphragm in, and then I'm not excited.

I feel weird about being excited. It seems not right, unless I ignore my judgements. Sex brings up feelings of being used sometimes. For a while, I felt very angry during sex because I felt used. The feelings were like old feelings of being forced or pressured into sex, and not saying "no".

How my Personal Lie affects my biggest problem with sex .... I can't have sex be satisfying and fun for me as a woman, and for my mate, because I'm a disappointment to myself and others as a woman.

Childhood incidents of sexuality .... My first experience with sex as a child was playing "doctor" with my girlfriends. I remember we would put our hands into each others' underpants, and I also remember not wanting to get caught, which we never did. This was in early grade school, I think. One person would be the doctor, and the other would lie in bed. The doctor would pass out pill candy, feel the patient, take her temperature, etc.

The other early experience of sexuality that I recall was after fourth grade and before eighth. It was when I saw a glimpse of my father's penis when he was wearing his pajamas one morning. When he sat down, the fly was open. I recall being curious, but not wanting to be found out looking. I said nothing and looked away fast. I also had the feeling I was seeing something I was not supposed to see, and I felt weird about it.

Church conditioning .... Sex was only OK in marriage, and a sin if done outside of marriage. People that had sex outside of marriage were bad and whores. (Stories of women in the Bible).

Parental conditioning .... I shouldn't have sex before I got married. When men came on to women, the women were "asking for it". My dad's implication was that the women were being flirts, or too sexy, and the men couldn't help themselves. Sex was never talked about openly. My mom never sat down and talked to me about sex. It was a taboo topic. I felt embarrassed watching people be romantic and kiss on TV when my parents were around.

My sister got pregnant out of marriage, when she was in college. It was a little hush-hush. She gave the baby up for adoption, and seemed to be still loved and accepted by my parents—although Dad was distant during that time, and Susie didn't feel comfortable being around him later. She was more comfortable with Dad when she got married, and the relationship really improved after they took the LRT together! I never got the idea sex was fun. I got more the feeling that it was something men wanted—and in some cases it was a duty. It was also something you didn't talk about.

Masturbation .... Aside from playing doctor in grade school, I don't recall masturbating for pleasure until in college, or maybe afterwards. I have faint recollections of touching myself around my clitoris, and it feeling tingly, but never of rubbing it to expand the feeling.

I started masturbating after having intercourse with men and not finding that particularly enjoyable. I never came either. I didn't even get involved in feeling the pleasure. If I did, I'd get excited, and then feel frustrated because I didn't climax.

So I started masturbating to see if I could climax, which I did. I initially felt a little guilty about masturbating. Sometimes I'd do it "secretly" after finishing intercourse, so I'd climax, but I never felt happy about that—just relieved and less frustrated. I never felt the climax was as real or totally enveloping as it would have been if I could come during intercourse.

19. DEBI

Conception description .... My father was angry—there was not enough sex for him. He also did not want a baby at that time. When he realized mom was pregnant, he wanted a boy.

How my conception affects my sexuality .... I picked up the thought from my dad at conception, "There is never enough sex". I feel angry about this issue. I have created this issue over and over again. I'm not having sex now. I am unwanted.

Also, my father wanted a boy. I am a girl. I thought that there was something wrong with me. I have spent most of my life wishing I was the opposite sex.

Birth description .... I was born in a Catholic Hospital. I was ready to come out, but the doctor wasn't there yet. The nurses and nuns wanted the doctor to be there, so they drugged us and crossed my mom's legs. In the struggle to get out, I wrapped the cord around my neck. I came out anyway, by myself. The doctor popped in, flung me around a little, and left.

How my birth affects my sexuality .... I feel unwanted sexually by men. I formed the thought that men are not there for me when I need them. I feel women hold me back and interfere in my relationships. I also have the thought that in an intimate relationship, I have to get out of there. My sexual experiences always seem to be too quick. The man never hangs around. He comes quickly, and I never get what I want.

I had a very quick and easy birth. Sex with my ex-husband was usually very quick and not satisfying. I felt like he was never really there for me. (Just like my obstetrician wasn't there.)

My Personal Lie is . . . . THERE IS SOMETHING WRONG WITH ME.

How my Personal Lie affects my sexuality . . . . I use this thought to avoid sex and relationships. I created the dis-ease, endometriosis. I created a situation to scar my body (which I still hate). I created an eating disorder to make myself overweight, so no one would want me. Since I became aware of my Personal Lie, I have lost thirty-five pounds, and the dis-ease is in the process of healing through rebirthing. (No doctors, no drugs, no more surgery.)

My biggest problem with sex is . . . . There is never enough.

My first memory of sexuality . . . . This was at about two months old. I was having my diaper changed by my father. He was playing with me and rubbing my vagina, and I really liked it.

Church conditioning . . . . I was raised Catholic, and sex was only allowed if you were going to have a baby. Sex was to be avoided otherwise. The nuns and priests at my school never talked about sex. If you were talking about sex you got in trouble.

Parental conditioning . . . . My parents never talked about sex until I was a teen, that I remember. They kept everything a big secret. Then my mom got out the book, showed me pictures, and told me lightly about sex. I made the decision then that it was disgusting, and I was never going to do it. That didn't last long.

Most embarrassing sexual situation . . . . I was masturbating on my door and my best friend came in. She teased me about it for years. I really thought that I was doing something wrong.

Childhood incident . . . . At five, my three-year-old brother was in the bathtub with me. I remember him licking me all over and I loved it. As the years went by, I had a lot of guilt about this time.

My Sexual Eternal Law is . . . . MY PERFECTION GIVES ME AN ABUNDANCE OF SEXUAL BLISS.

20. JOY

Conception description . . . . My conception happened at my grandmother's house, in the bed my mother had slept in as a child. My father had been away at sea for nine months. When he got back, he and mom decided it was time to have a child. I was conceived right away.

How my conception affects my sexuality . . . . If I knew a man wanted me, I would have sex with him right away. After my husband and I had been married a little over nine months, we went and lived with my parents for a while. I always felt real safe making love in my parents' home. A thought I had at my conception was it was a mistake to be in a body, and a mistake to have sex with many, many partners. I always had the thought that I was making a mistake.

Birth description . . . . I was born three weeks early. My parents were expecting a boy, and I was a girl. My obstetrician decided Mom would be in labor another three or four hours, so he left and another doctor came in and delivered me. I felt unwanted by my original obstetrician.

How my birth affects my sexuality . . . . I felt wrong and unwanted as a woman.

My Personal Lie . . . . I AM WRONG AND UNWANTED AS A WOMAN.

How my Personal Lie affects my sexuality . . . . I create men not wanting me. I've created issues with my husband when I thought he wanted to do lots of other things besides make love with me when I wanted to. During lovemaking, I've had anger come up about not feeling I could be the initiator, or come on strong. Feeling that if I were a man, I could.

My biggest problem with sex . . . . I don't get sex when I want it. I was fed on a schedule, and knew that I couldn't get what I wanted. I have orgasms, but not vaginally.

How my Personal Lie affects my biggest problem with sex . . . . Since I'm unwanted and wrong as a woman, my thoughts are that "I don't get what I want", and "The way I have orgasms is wrong", and "If I were a man, I'd get what I want".

21. DIANA

Conception description .... I felt unplanned and unwanted, because my parents didn't consciously want to conceive a child. My mother was using contraception (a cervical cap). I also feel my parents were feeling very separate from each other in their lovemaking. My mother's thoughts about sex were that it was emotionally very painful, and that she felt really impatient for it to be over and done with. My father's thought was that it was inevitable that he hurt women. It feels like there was a lot of sadness in him as well.

How my conception affects my sexuality .... I've always resented using any form of contraception. I feel that sex in relationships has to be emotionally painful. I feel like it's inevitable that I'm hurt by the men I'm attracted to. In the past, I have vacillated between being very sexually active, and being totally shut down.

I have tried to create intimacy through sex, and have blamed my sexuality when relationships broke up. I create feeling either used or rejected. I either love making love and feel spiritually connected, or I hate it and feel it intrudes on intimacy. I feel at the effect of planned sex, and need a lot of emotional reassurance and play to feel innocent about it. It feels easier to have planned sex if I'm a bit drugged. I feel trapped and smothered by sex in committed relationships, so I create being used or rejected. Then I can leave, and prove that sex creates separation.

Birth description .... My father wasn't present at my birth, so I felt unwanted in my body as a female. I feel my mother would rather have had a boy, for my father's sake. My labor was about a week late, and lasted eleven hours. My mother was anesthetized prior to my delivery, and they pulled me out with forceps. My face was very bruised, and I felt roughly handled. My bottom was smacked by the doctor.

I was born in a small country hospital at visiting time, and my birth kept all the visitors waiting, because all the staff were at my delivery. I feel I must have been rotated with forceps prior to delivery.

How my birth affects my sexuality .... I'm the eldest child, so I felt unwanted as a female by my mother, and bought into the thought that women should always be thinking about what men want. I often feel uncertainty about timing and sex, and won't initiate it when I feel like it. When lovemaking goes on for too long, I can feel impatient for it to end. I feel unconscious around completing sexually. I rarely experience vaginal orgasms, because I feel powerless, and at the effect of men. I think that if I don't go along with what men want, the relationship will become violent. I hate men spanking me while I'm making love. My timing in sex and relationships is inconvenient. I notice I go round in circles, and want men to pull me out of the pattern.

22. PATTY

Conception description .... My mom didn't like sex. I don't believe she's ever had an orgasm. She didn't like being touched. (My dad had sweaty, clammy hands.) Sex was a wifely duty to be performed, but not enjoyed. My mom had been suicidal five months before I was conceived, and I knew she hadn't gotten her life together in that time. So I asked how I came into the picture, and she said it wasn't planned—it was a mistake. She and my dad had gone out and got snockered, and they forgot to use anything.

How my conception affects my sexuality .... In the past, I really didn't care for sex. My body didn't feel, and my relationships suffered for it. I was good at giving to others so I wouldn't have to receive. I picked takers so I wouldn't receive. Then when I felt safe enough to receive, it was too bad, because I hadn't picked a person who was a giver.

When I was in a relationship long enough for the person to want to give to me, I just didn't know how to receive. The last person I was involved with had a lot of expectations, like a man. Success was equal to orgasm. I was feeling more, and liking to be touched, but that wasn't enough. When I would express what I wanted, she felt I was putting her down. There was no intimacy. It was her way or not at all, so for a long time it was not at all.

Birth description .... I had a female doctor. I was separated from my mother immediately after birth, and left in the hospital for two weeks. When I got home, I couldn't be around my mom for five or six more weeks, because she had the mumps.

How my birth affects my sexuality .... Perhaps I seek out love, affection and intimacy from women because I didn't get it at birth.

My Personal Lie .... I AM THE OPPOSITE. I AM THE WRONG SEX, AND NOT WANTED BECAUSE OF IT.

How my Personal Lie affects my sexuality .... I have a lot of opposites in my life. Sexually, I seek out women, and society says it should be men.

My biggest problem with sex is . . . . Letting my femininity shine, and being safe in my vulnerability to feel and receive.

How my Personal Lie affects my biggest problem is sex is . . . . I have thought myself to have sexual dyslexia. The normal way is maleness gives, femaleness receives. I have been a female giver, but not a very good receiver. As I feel more comfortable in my femininity, I am enjoying the rewards of receiving, and am finding myself to be stronger as I'm more vulnerable.

Childhood incidents of sexuality . . . . I was about four years old when the earliest one I can remember happened. My aunt and uncle had a ranch, and I was visiting them. My cousin and I wanted to ride horses, so I walked up to the saddle house to ask my cousin's grandfather to saddle the horses for us. The next thing I remember is his hands in my pants. I don't know if he just touched me, or entered me. He asked me if it felt good. I was not allowed to say "no" to my parents or other adults, so I was afraid to say "no." I said "yes," knowing that I meant "no." Later when I discussed this with my father, he said he wanted to teach us to respect adults—it was not that we couldn't say "no." Although he did think a child who said "no" didn't respect adults.

The next incident I remember was in kindergarten. I don't remember much about kindergarten except this experience. I wore a dress to school one day. We were sitting on the floor, and a little Mexican boy sat behind me with his hands in my pants. Again, I had a feeling of being frozen, and not saying "Don't do that!" I don't ever remember wearing a dress after that.

Masturbation . . . . I never masturbated. I never got touched when I was born, and my family wasn't affectionate, so I didn't know that touching myself could feel good. I feel like I grew up asexual—with sex not being a part of my life. When I was about twenty-seven, a partner introduced me to a vibrator. That was actually the first time I realized that I wasn't totally dead, and that I could actually experience sexual feelings.

Church conditioning . . . . I grew up in the Presbyterian Church, and was involved in a Christian youth group in high school and junior college. I don't remember much being said about sex, except that you were not supposed to be sexual before marriage, and that you take Christ into everything you do. I didn't feel safe from boys even in church. We would go down as a group to Disneyland in the church bus, and the guys wanted to get the girls in the back of the bus, to mess around, or to show they had a girlfriend.

Parental conditioning . . . . I don't remember my parents ever saying anything about sex. I didn't date, or ever have a boy friend, so they didn't have anything to worry about, I guess.

Embarrassing sexual situation . . . . I got myself into the same kind of situation when I was a sophomore or junior in high school, as I had been in when I was four or five on my uncle's ranch. I was at the drive-in with a friend and her mother. She was there to meet her boyfriend, because her father wouldn't let her see him. When her boyfriend got in the car, his friend asked if I wanted to sit with him. I was still trying to convince myself I liked guys, so I said OK. It was in the cab of a truck, and he had a male friend in there, so it was rather crowded. I wanted this guy to put his arm around me, and so I did some deep breathing, rubbing my breast on his arm. He thought I wanted him to fondle my breast, so he put his arm around me and started squeezing my breast. There I was frozen again, not able to say "stop." I wanted to get out of there, but I couldn't move. Finally, I got enough nerve to say I wanted out, and I left.

23. SALLY

Conception description . . . . My parents really felt uncomfortable about sex or sexuality in public—everything was real under cover. I feel Mom often felt that sex was what a woman should do, almost that it was a service to the man.

How my conception affects my sexuality . . . . I attract men who can't show love in public—even holding hands. I feel I can't ask for what I want. I feel I should satisfy the man, and I come second.

Birth description . . . . I was not the sex my father wanted, and he was not at my birth. My mother was worried about the health of my grandmother, and this made my environment feel unsafe. I was induced to come early. My labor was long, and a struggle.

How my birth affects my sexuality . . . . In my first relationship, I fought my partner all the way in order to retain my virginity, and then I lost it all in a rush at the end. I often think things over for ages, and then feel I have to act now, or rather, yesterday. I feel a great urgency once I decide something, I do it quickly.

I feel I'm not good enough for me or my partner. I can't really let myself go sexually—I'm always thinking my partners will compare me with other women. I don't feel comfortable as a woman.

I have to prove all the time that I'm better than a woman; that I'm good enough to be a man. I had more men friends than women for a while. Men aren't really there for me. I feel I'm being used. They are just there for their pleasure. I'm not getting what I want for me. Often men will turn their backs on me after sex, or go for a glass of water and go to sleep. They hardly ever cuddle. I can't get what I want when I want it. They never talk and ask how I really feel. One boyfriend made me lie on my stomach all the way through sex—I felt really used.

My first memory of sexuality .... When I was about three or four, I discovered my genitals and began to masturbate. Mom would hit my hands, or push them away. When I persisted, she would tie my hands behind my back.

My cousin and I inspected ourselves when young. He was my age, and later he wanted to see what I looked like, and tried to pull my swimsuit off. I attacked him, and was reprimanded for scratching him. I never told anyone why I protected myself.

Parental conditioning .... I was told, no sex outside of marriage. There were no jokes or public shows of love. Mom showed us a book on sex and our sex organs, and then shut down when we asked, "How do you do it?"

Most embarrassing sexual experience .... A boyfriend got excited, and had a premature ejaculation on me in the bed. Embarrassing for us both.

First sexual experience .... It was with my ex-fiancee when I was eighteen. I fought him, and held off from having sex with him for six months, before giving in. I felt a real relief when it was over. There wasn't all that much to it anyway. I wanted so much to please him. I felt I gave my power away to him.

My Personal Lie is .... I'M NOT GOOD ENOUGH.

How my Personal Lie affects my sexuality .... I feel guilty for being a woman and not a man. No wonder I'm a hermit. I use my job as an excuse not to go out and meet new people. Men may reject me, or I may not measure up to their standards.

My biggest problem with sex is . . . . Men use sex to control me. I feel that I have to give it as payment eventually. Why do men have sex always on their minds!?

How my Personal Lie affects my biggest problem with sex . . . . I'm bad, not good enough, so I will never have a warm, loving, totally satisfying lover who will think of me as a person with my own needs.

24. CONNIE

Conception description . . . . My primary thought is that love hurts. I feel that my dad used sex as a weapon, and an access point to feeling alive. He was an up-and-coming accountant looking for further training in law. It's a belief in our family that he named me in order to get his family's wealth. Dad's hearing was affected by the war, and about that time I think his dermatitis began to appear.

A believer in the roles of men and women, he agreed that women where only good for two things—to be underneath a man or look after the home. He was very connected to his mother, who was a dominating, strong-willed woman—surviving her husband who had been sick since the war. My mother's family was wealthy, but lost in the depression. She remains bitter about this. Dad, I believe, had a lot of unresolved issues. He was trying for inherited wealth rather than earned. (A dynamic still operating in our family.)

I'm sure my dad liked sex, but felt guilty about it. I think he felt guilty about hurting my mother, who, being the submissive type, did what he ordered. He later married a strong-willed woman, and I felt he blossomed in that relationship. Mom, I feel, was oppressed by Dad, as she also believed and maintained the strict roles (stereotypes).

She tells me that sex with him was good, and that he often wouldn't wait until she had her diaphragm in. I feel that both of them thought sex was a duty. I've felt that mom had the thought of feeling guilty about liking sex and liking it rough.

Mom tells me that she knew she'd married the wrong man pretty soon into the marriage. They had three older children—boy, girl, girl—and wanted another boy to even it up. I'm sure they both wanted a boy—Dad particularly, as Tony was proving not to be the macho man's dream of a son.

It was three and a half years of trying to conceive, which mom is constantly amazed at, as all of the other pregnancies before and after seemed to fly in.

I feel that Mom particularly wanted me to hold the family together, to hold Dad's attention. She says he loved the babies, but couldn't cope when they were saying "no," or talking and questioning.

How my conception affects my sexuality .... I think my conception thoughts were, "Love hurts," "My role is to help heal family tension," "I'm not wanted as a girl," "I'm not enough (as a girl) to do this, it's too much for me."

I have chosen partners that seem to need help in getting in touch with themselves and communicating. Who are somehow not fully able to function, or are disadvantaged.

I doubt that I am ever wanted, as I have always been the initiator. I have been quite good at listening, advising, soothing and comforting. Not expressing my needs—just feeling uncomfortable, which builds to a total frustration, and then I leave.

I often hold myself back, feeling that if I don't, I'll be too much and overpower my partner. Then he'll reject me. This has often been said to me, "You're just too much." I give, and have difficulty relaxing when being given to, not believing the man really wants me to enjoy it.

Birth description .... The cord was around my neck. My birth was fast, and I feel I was probably held back. Mom was drugged and Dad was in bed (I think).

How my birth affects my sexuality .... I feel like I move very fast, create an obstacle, and then struggle. I sabotage myself a lot with feelings of doubt, feelings that I'm not good enough, or that it'll be too much for me or that I can't.

In the expression of my sexuality, I have often moved very quickly into bed rather than getting to know the man intimately. (Although mostly I sleep with people I've known for a while.) I often want to go very fast and space out a bit. Going hard and fast, and not allowing enough time for me to receive, has often led to sex being over too soon, with me feeling ripped off.

Incest with father .... That is the dynamic I felt with my father. Most of the flashbacks I've had about having sex with him have come during sex. Some very frightening and some releasing, like this one: "Oh, this is what he did too—that was then and not nice, this is not and is."

There were about seven to eight years of incest with my Dad. I've remembered him throwing me on to his bed and lying on me. Squeezing my legs together so they clasped around his penis, his weight forward on my upper body. I felt smashed and terrified of suffocation.

The energy in my body felt too much and unsafe. I'm sure it was a part of my hyperactivity (which I dulled out with T.V.). I have often had the sense that the energy in my body is too much. I feel that I still jump around and fidget. I know I use exercise to move it about.

It seems that I have spent a long time waiting for my father to come and take me away with him. Most of my lovers have "been" him and I have felt betrayed by him after.

When he died while I was in India, I was "out of control" with grief and rage. No one in the family wanted to hear me. It was my experience, my way of seeing how much he meant to me.

Dad's gift to me, I feel, is inner strength and deep loving. At times I "get it," at other times I flatly "don't."

Puberty .... After Mom and us girls left Dad unexpectedly when I was thirteen or fourteen, I began masturbating, which I did a lot. It always seemed wrong, and not the right way. As it was more of a clitoral rub, I would masturbate on things—pillows in particular and I didn't need to undress. It become very furtive and there was something I enjoyed about it being so. Around this time, sometimes I would finger my anus—often until it bled. Sometimes with the thought of helping out stuck bits of shit. I'm unclear as to why I did this. It has a peculiar charge for me which I feel is surfacing. Even now I felt slightly that it's not OK, that it's the wrong way, and that I could be re-creating Dad's fucking style.

My first teenage sexual experience .... That I remember was with a boy I met at a party. Within minutes, we were lying on the parents' bedroom floor, his fingers inside me, saying this isn't working, it's not right. Although not really knowing what was going on, I concluded yet again that there was something wrong with me, that I wasn't what I should be.

I lost my virginity to a twenty-seven year old man when I was sixteen, I told Mom, got on the pill, and had sex arranged, in control. I became the knowing one, the giver, the turner on. I didn't bleed, which I was expecting. I could not touch his penis with my hands. I told him I was scared, and that something had happened in my past (what, I didn't know.)

I've slept with around fifteen to twenty men, and five women. I lived with a man from when I was eighteen to twenty-three. Then I left and started having relationships with women. The first night I slept with a woman, I had a dream of sleeping with my father. It wasn't until two years later that I began having rememberances—flashbacks of incest experiences.

25. SUE

Conception description .... My parents wanted a boy to carry on the family name, as my dad was an only son. My mother's thoughts about sex were that it was disgusting, dirty, and a chore that women had to perform to keep their husbands. If you enjoyed it, you were bad and guilty. My mother felt a lot of shame about her body, and wasn't present consciously during my conception, either from drinking, or from just being out of her body. My parents had very strong thoughts that what they were doing was wrong.

How my conception affects my sexuality .... I usually am out of my body, or very stoned, when I have sex. I also have a lot of shame about my body, and usually prefer to have sex in the dark, with only a candle lit, or a very small light. I feel that sex, when there's the possibility of "getting caught," is very exciting. I feel like it's wrong to want sex or feel turned on, so I am attracted to men who I feel safe flirting with, like married men or gay men. I know I'll never act out my desires with them. My thoughts about being wrong caused me to create myself the wrong sex.

Birth description .... I was born via a caesarean. My labor was long, and I was drugged. The obstetrician who delivered me knew how much my parents wanted a boy, so the first thing he said to my dad was "I'm sorry to tell you this, but it is a girl." I was a disappointment as a girl.

How my birth affects my sexuality .... I've always felt very wrong as a woman. I've never felt feminine, or like I could be really sexually attractive. I was always a tomboy, and tried very hard to be the son my dad never had. I went everywhere with him. I went hunting and fishing, and was always very good at sports. I have lots of claustrophobia about sleeping facing my partner and in his embrace. I'm never able to sleep in the nude because of my shame about my body. I jump up immediately, and put on a nightgown or pajamas.

I've always had a problem about having people waiting for me to have pleasure sexually. I'm very frustrated if we don't make love fast. I like fast, intense lovemaking with lots of kissing and hugging and cuddling. Most of the time I feel like I'd rather do that then the actual act of making love. I love parking and necking. Because I feel like sex is dirty, I always like to put a towel under both of us, and have tissues or a washcloth handy, so the sheets don't get messed up. I jump up right away and go wash myself off or douche. I don't really like oral sex. I don't mind performing it for my partner, but really hate him doing it to me.

Since I was drugged at birth, I like to be stoned or high to make love. Sometimes I resent my partner, because I feel like because he's the man and

I'm a woman, I owe it to him to have sex whether I want to or not: that his needs are more important than mine. I've done a lot of things in bed that I felt were disgusting, because I was supposed to please my partner. It seems as if my body doesn't even belong to me. My parents didn't have a lot of money at the time I was born, so I have the thought that men only want me for sex or money. I've always felt too guilty to allow myself to have many orgasms, so sex almost always leaves me unsatisfied and disappointed.

Puberty . . . . I remember the day I got my first bra. My mother and her mother decided it was time I should wear one, at about age twelve. After they made me put it on, I was so full of rage and dismay that I couldn't be one of the boys anymore, that I went outside and broke the straps off so I wouldn't have to wear it. My grandmother sewed them up, and I had to put it back on. To this day I hate bras. I really resent wearing them, and no matter how much weight I gain, my breasts seem to stay small. If I diet and lost weight, the first area to go is my breasts.

I remember getting my first period somewhere around age thirteen. Mom had never told me about menstruation, and I felt a lot of fear and shame about it. To this day, I get very embarrassed if I think men can tell I'm having my period. I think having sex while I'm menstruating is very disgusting. I've always felt guilt about being a woman—I create partners who are insensitive and abuse me to varying degrees.

Sexual relationships . . . . Something else I've become aware of, is how the universe has supported me in getting off my judgements about people who are very sexual, especially topless dancers and prostitutes. I created having my first husband leave me for a topless dancer. The next partner I had that I lived with, had a best friend whose mate was a topless dancer. We moved next door to them, and she became my best friend for a long time. She really helped me enjoy my sexuality, and I feel that was the time of my life when I looked the best and had the most fun.

Then I became attracted to my husband, who during his drug-dealing days, spent a lot of time in topless bars selling drugs. Once, when we'd separated for a few days, I came back to pick up some boots, and caught him in bed with a woman who's a topless dancer.

Last year in the Bahamas, I created being roommates with a wonderful woman from Anchorage who is a "dancing rebirther." We became very close, and she taught me a lot about sexuality and innocence.

I see now that I've always been plugged in by sexually overt (flagrant) people. This is to heal my thoughts about sex not being innocent.

26. LOIS

Birth description . . . . My mother's fears were very intense for two months preceeding my birth. My father was in England during the war, and she was afraid he would be killed, or that he would stay there with a woman he wrote he was having an affair with. He was not at my birth.

I did not see my father until I was fourteen months old, and well past my initial birth trauma, and had been healed of the infantile paralysis I had at six months of age. I believe the paralysis was due to a birth injury which caused my left leg to be limp and lifeless for two months. This was a significant factor in my dad's decision to return to my mother. I was supposed to become a cripple.

My birth was a face presentation. A type of breech birth, with intense pain, struggle, and confusion, due to coming out wrong, and being the wrong sex. My mother had had a miscarriage two years before me that was a boy, and I sense it was me.

The doctor was angry and swearing, "This is all wrong." He pulled at my collar bone, and shoulders, then at my rib cage, as I was stuck at the pelvic area, and the cord was pulled tight and pinched. I was breathing on my own, as my chest and stomach were free, and feeling very confused about all the action. The doctor was intensely focused on the cord, and seemed panicked to get me out. My mom's labor was long and hard. She was given anesthesia earlier, and this just made it slow and difficult, as she was holding back due to fear.

When I finally got out the doctor cut my cord. He was so absorbed in his panic that he neglected to notice that I was already breathing. He grabbed me hard at the ankles, jerked me up and hit me on the bottom so hard I felt a jolt go through my whole body. My mother expressed that my dad would be disappointed that I was a girl. Then they took me away from my mom, and I felt I was not wanted, or that something was wrong with me or my mom. I just felt lost and confused.

How my birth affects my sexuality . . . . In taking on my mother's fears of losing daddy and trying to raise my sister and I alone, I made a mental promise to be responsible to help save their marriage.

I carry this into my relationships and assume all the responsibility or guilt if things are not working. I go overboard to try and please my partner, make sure he is satisfied, and let him know he has satisfied me. I always feel real sensitive to the male ego, and feel responsible if they are expressing the least bit of unhappiness. This is connected to my dad always expressing his unhappiness that mother never enjoyed sex, and my thought that this is why he wanted someone else.

My father not being at my birth, and this being partly due to his wanting to be with another woman, seems to have a very strong effect on my relationships. In the majority of my relationships men have not been there for me as a real friend, they have been there for sex.

The two men I married seemed to enjoy sex, and being catered to and served. This felt real natural for me to do with my southern, submissive upbringing, but I felt alone and rejected when I was in need of a friend I could talk to. I always felt I was a disappointment to them if I could not handle everything on my own, especially if it was emotional in any way.

The number eight has been a significant timing pattern for me. I believe this started in the eighth month of pregnancy with the fear of my father not returning.

When I was eight years old, my father had incest with my older sister. After this, he pushed me away, due to the strain he and mom felt trying to work it out and stay together. I didn't know what was going on then, I just felt rejected, as I was not allowed to sit on his lap, and he withdrew all affection from me. I felt the change was due to something going on with mom and my sister as everyone was so tense and angry all the time.

At sixteen, my dad and I had the worst time getting along. I found out about the incest and was afraid to be alone with him. My sister was married, but came home with her husband to live with us. My dad always compared me to her, yelled at me for everything, hit me upside my head if I expressed any kind of disagreement, called me a no-good idiot all the time, and just in general made my life miserable. I rebelled, started smoking, quit school, and got married to get away from him.

At 24, my marriage broke up. The catalytic agent was my husband's affair with one of my best friends. I totally rebelled after our divorce, and sowed my wild oats in an effort to get even, and to prove to myself I was good enough in bed and in general, good enough to make it on my own.

At approximately 32, I got married again. At approximately 40, I ended my second marriage. As you can guess, another woman was a significant factor in my decision to leave. I never felt I was good enough to win my father's approval, and have consistently set up the same patterns of rejection with other men in order to prove my thoughts are right.

It seems I am either overcompensating by going all out to please and to prove how good I am, or going in the opposite direction and disappointing other's expectations of me. I do this by letting them down, running away or rebelling, or getting angry and going into isolation with an attitude of "I can do it myself, I don't need you and I won't let you hurt me".

Face presentation shows up as men expressing how different I am than what they expected me to be. For instance, they seem surprised I am as open, aware, responsive, and experienced as I am, for they say I look so straight-laced, controlled, or like that. Others tell me that they perceive the energy I put out as so powerfully sexy that they are surprised when I get indignant at them when they come on strong. I guess coming out opposite and confused about my sexuality causes me to put out mixed messages.

I also have a real headstrong right/wrong issue, and defensiveness about being told I'm wrong. A rebellious attitude—especially with men whom I perceive as being real macho or authoritative. Thank God I am softening on all of that. I also have a very direct, head-on, face-forward type of approach, which seems to threaten or turn off a lot of men. I have been told consistently by male and female friends to stifle my aliveness and intelligence and to tone it down, to take a more subtle approach to get what I want from a man. This feels phony and manipulative to me, but I have become much more easy going and quieter after doing rebirthing.

Oedipal period . . . . Pain, struggle and confusion at my birth set up thought patterns of same. My first sexual experience was with an uncle who tried to play with me when I was five years old. It hurt because his hands were rough and he was not gentle, yet it also felt somewhat pleasant. I felt this was very bad and wrong to do, and I was scared to tell anyone and afraid of being hurt. I just felt so confused and scared to tell him not to touch me.

But my uncle told me it was OK to let him touch me because he loved me, and it was OK for me to love him that way. I felt wrong to say "yes", and afraid to hurt his feelings if I said "no". I was sensitive to the male ego even then, but so afraid of hurt, guilt and shame that I started to cry. I think he was afraid I would tell, so he stopped and said it was OK, but not to tell.

This pattern repeated two other times. As I got older, I would let boys kiss me and hold me close and neck, but I always stopped out of fear and confusion. I was a good girl who said "no" due to my fear of getting a bad reputation, or that it would ruin me and no one would want me for a wife. I liked feeling sexual though, and masturbated a lot, even though I thought this was bad too.

When I got married, I still felt confused and guilty about sex, but I enjoyed it a lot. I could not reach a climax with normal penetration for the first two years of my marriage because I always got real sore before my husband could satisfy me. His penis hurt me, but I liked his hand. I could climax with his hand, so I felt guilty for masturbating, as I thought this had somehow spoiled me, and now I couldn't do it right with normal penetration. My husband felt bad about not being able to satisfy me, and all the reassuring in the world did not seem to ease his frustration. This just added to my guilt, as I felt responsible for his feelings and his ego.

This situation improved after the birth of our first child, and we really started to enjoy our sex life. We loved to grab quickies whenever we could find a few moments away from the kids.

In conclusion, I have played out my birth thoughts and my Personal Lies, such as SOMETHING IS WRONG WITH ME, I CAN'T DO IT RIGHT, I'M NOT GOOD ENOUGH AS A WOMAN, etc. all my life, in all areas of my life, but especially in my relationships with men and in my relationship with my body, i.e. through overweight, illness and injury.

These thoughts have caused me to overcompensate in my reactions to situations in my relationships. I have spent most of my sexually active years so far trying hard to learn, stretch, grow, give more, and perform at my best, all in an effort to prove to men (to myself in reality), that I AM A GOOD WOMAN. I guess I thought this would prevent the dreaded rejection-for-another-woman pattern. I realize now that I keep setting this up because of my birth thoughts. My mind wants to be right. Well guess what? I AM WILLING TO BE WRONG ABOUT ALL OF THESE THOUGHTS! THIS IS NOT REAL! I am willing to accept the truth that I AM PERFECTLY RIGHT AS I AM IN EACH AND EVERY MOMENT. THANK YOU, GOD.

27. GLENDA

Birth description . . . . Forceps & drugs.

How my birth affects my sexuality . . . . Because of my forceps birth, I'm always waiting for someone to "pull me out". I'm waiting for someone to make the moves sexually with me first. As long as they are having a good time then that's OK. As for me, I'm still waiting.

My Personal Lie is . . . . I'M NOT GOOD ENOUGH AND THERE'S SOMETHING WRONG WITH ME.

How my Personal Lie affects my sexuality . . . . I'm not allowing myself to have what I want. By holding myself back, I get to reinforce "I'm not good enough . . . " and especially " . . . there's something wrong with me". Because if I were OK, I would have good sex. Because I'm not OK, I don't have good sex.

Important: The one and only time I have had incredible, fantastic orgasms continuously all night was when I was very high on marijuana (very strong stuff from Venezuela). I was with a very close, old friend, and we both got ripped out of our minds. It was the best sex in my whole life. My mind was somewhere; I was definitely not my normal self in bed. I could hardly move, it was just happening to me. I'll never forget that.

Parental conditioning .... No one mentioned sex in our family, especially my mother and father. I got lots of "warnings" from my mother that "Men are only after one thing," "Men get girls into trouble," "Watch out for those bad men," and "Men are bad!" My mother didn't really say anything to me about how babies were born. I went to the library to find out when I was eleven and older. I had heard all my girlfriends talk about sex and babies, so I did some research myself. Sex was this big mystery to me, something you did not talk about.

Masturbation .... I did not masturbate as a child as far as I can remember. I remember all sorts of feelings I would get—but I never really masturbated as such. I might have touched myself from time to time, in bed, late at night, hidden under the covers.

Church conditioning .... There was no real church conditioning as our family was not religious. I only went to Sunday School until I was 5 years old. My parents were very old-fashioned though—no one knew how to communicate.

Sexual history .... When I first started dating I was very "frigid". I would not let anyone have sexual intercourse with me. I let some boyfriends touch me, but only so far. I had no real sexual feelings at that time, just an incredible wall up between myself and any man. I was incredibly shy around men. I found it hard to talk to them, and had no self-confidence.

My first act of actual sexual intercourse was horrible. I had let some boyfriends (I never had anyone steady) go so far, but was still a virgin until I was three days short of being seventeen. I had a crush on this blond guy who hung around in our group. His name was Les, and he was a ladies' man. I liked him a lot. We went out together and he took me home. He made love to me in the front seat of the car. I remember how much it hurt. I bled later. I didn't really know what was happening; I was so naive in those days. Anyway, it was most unpleasant for me.

Later I found out to my embarrassment that he gave me "crabs". I had to take care of that without telling anyone. I never saw him again. I was deeply hurt. Since then I have had a lot of sexual experiences. For most of them, I have needed some drink or drugs to make me feel sexy. A lot of times I've waited for the other person to make the moves. I have never really asked for what I want. I just expect the other person to know. I don't orgasm with a man during sexual intercourse.

When I lived in London, eight years ago, I took a woman's group which was for women who had never had an orgasm. I learned that lots of women can only orgasm by being stimulated on the clitoris. They gave us vibrators and books, and we went home and practised. That was the first time I can remember masturbating. I was around 25. That helped me a lot because after that I met a guy who I managed to have clitoral orgasms with. He seemed to know what I needed, because I never really asked him. He wouldn't give up, and wanted to please me. Since then I haven't asked for what I want.

I've taken several workshops on sensuality and sexuality, and I feel a bit hopeless. My attitude is (or I should say, my thoughts are), is "As long as the man is OK, it doesn't really bother me", "Sex is not the most important thing, as long as I've got a man", "I'm too embarrassed to ask for what I want", "I'm waiting for him to do what I like, whatever that is", "It's hopeless anyway".

28. GARY

Conception description . . . . My parents' thoughts about sex are that it is just for making children, and that having children is a struggle. My mother had two miscarriages before me.

How my conception affects my sexuality . . . . I feel like it's really not OK to have sex just for fun sometimes. It's just for making children. This is not a common occurrence though. I have a strong feeling that it's a struggle to have children. I worry about women getting pregnant. My mother thought, "I can't have children"—she had two miscarriages before me.

Birth description . . . . I was a forceps delivery. At the time of my birth, I did not receive my mother's love.

How my birth affects by sexuality . . . . I like to be controlled sexually and manually manipulated. I want the woman to take control of the whole process. I often will just let her masturbate me and not want to make love to her. All my relationships, including fourteen years of marriage, were set up to create sexual manipulation to echo the manipulation by my obstetrician with the forceps. I married when I was 21, and moved straight from home to marriage. I attracted other women into my marriage, and always wanted women outside of my marriage.

My biggest problem with sex is .... The hook-up between sex for pleasure and sex to procreate. Having experienced the height of ecstasy in sexual bliss, I now would like to realize this blissful state without the need for sex. (This applies to my primary relationship.) For other relationships, my biggest problem would be a fear of not being good enough, not being able to satisfy my partner and not being able to make love as long as she may desire—length of time per session, and number of sessions in a night.

My Personal Lie .... is I AM WEAK. It makes me feel weak and inadequate with a strong, powerful woman. I am always afraid when making love for the first time that I won't be good enough, and that I will be compared to previous lovers. I therefore try hard to please the woman, and often forget about myself.

My first memory of sexuality .... Was the strange feelings I got when I looked at the glass suction cup my mother used to help her breastfeed my brother. I was probably between five and seven.

Church conditioning .... Up until I left the Presbyterian Church at fifteen, I have no recollection of sex and sexuality even being discussed at Sunday school or in sermons.

Parental conditioning .... I was never told anything, except for a vague discussion with Dad, just before I got married at twenty-one. My observation of my parents was that close body contact, and showing love for each other in public, was not normal. I never saw them make love—they would shut the bedroom door sometimes and I never knew why.

Most embarrassing sexual situations .... As a teenager I had general feelings of embarrassment about sex when I heard others talking about things I didn't understand. I thought everyone knew more about it and had done more than me. I felt inadequate—buying condoms!

As an adult my most embarrassing situation in sex was when I couldn't get an erection. I tried three times with one woman just after I separated from my wife, and I would lose my erection right at the moment of penetration. She was quite inexperienced compared to me, and yet I had feelings of being weak and totally inadequate as a man. This is perhaps related to my belief that my penis is too small, and that I'm being compared to others.

My first sexual experience with intercourse .... I was seventeen, and it occurred at my girl friend's parents' house while they were away on holidays. She and her older brother were looking after themselves.

I felt scared and yet extremely excited and in love. She was a virgin, and I was worried about what would happen when the hymen broke. We put a towel down on the bed in case there was a lot of blood. In actual fact, there was not much and it was quite easy.

I don't even remember if she climaxed, probably not. But we both enjoyed it, and decided to keep doing it and learning more about sex. I didn't use a condom, and had to pull out before ejaculating.

29. DIANE

Birth description . . . . I had a fast birth—three or four hours. I was held back, waiting for the obstetrician. He made it there half way through the delivery. My father was not at my delivery. Gas was given to my mother, and I was separated from her. The delivery was normal.

Decisions . . . .

1. I can't have what I want.
2. I'm out of control.
3. It's not safe to be alive and powerful as a woman.
4. I'm trapped.
5. I have to do it on my own or without men.
6. There must be something wrong with me.
7. I'm dirty.
8. I'm guilty.
9. I hurt people.
10. I'm separate from the source.
11. I'm separate.
12. I'm not important.
13. Life is a struggle.

How my birth affects my sexuality . . . I often feel I want sex fast and passionate. If this doesn't happen, my passion dies and I feel frustrated, cheated and angry. If my partner wants to play around for a long time, I feel held back, sometimes bored, and start going unconscious: "I can't have what I want." I feel anesthetized.

I created recurrent yeast infections so I felt "dirty" and "contagious" and "guilty" about having sex: "I can't have what I want." I created something wrong with me.

I notice I hold back my enjoyment of orgasm for fear of being seen to be out of control: "It's not safe to be alive and powerful as a woman." I often feel boring and uninteresting, especially in the company of men: "I'm not important."

I often want to go unconscious when I get into bed, even though I also feel like having sex. I feel overwhelmed by tiredness—this could be related to the anesthesia my mother received during my labor.

I feel I have guilt about being separate from God, or the source. I feel guilty about having a body and enjoying my body: "I don't want to be here". I have a habit of going unconscious in life in general, and especially during sex.

During my relationship with my husband, I often felt very separate from him because he was only physically with me, not spiritually. This turned me off to sex with him.

I have a fear of being "trapped" in my relationships. I believe that I have to do things on my own or without men. That it's not safe to be supported, because then I would be vulnerable and out of control. I feel that to have what I want, I have to be in control, and do it all myself. I manifested this by taking on the burdens of running the household and working full time, and often financially supporting my partner.

I also have a thought that I am physically annoying, or that I hurt men. I notice myself thinking that I am too heavy if I'm lying or sitting on them, or that they don't like it when I touch them. I believe I caused my husband a lot of emotional pain when we separated.

I also have the feeling of being held back in my relationships. I believe I can't follow my true passion because it would lead to separation. That I would be too overwhelming and powerful and men wouldn't like it (i.e. the obstetrician).

30. EVE

Conception description . . . . My father felt angry at my mother for making him feel bad about himself. He was sick of her. My mother was shut down but angry—felt she didn't have a choice at that time. I experienced it as becoming enclosed in darkness. Being swallowed up and losing myself.

How my conception affects my sexuality .... I find strong male energy attractive. I think men don't care about me and are just into their own stuff, but I will be there for them anyway, whether I feel like it or not. I think I will lose them If I'm not there for them, or invite their anger. I am unable to feel much, probably because I am suppressing anger and sadness. I do this because of my belief that I don't matter enough, and my fear of losing myself if I surrendered.

Birth description .... I felt betrayed by my mother at birth. I had felt safe and warm inside her, but after I was born she wasn't there for me so much anymore. I didn't understand it—where she had gone. I felt betrayed because I had trusted her with my complete vulnerability, and now her energy was gone. I felt alone and frightened.

How my birth affects my sexuality .... In sex, I find myself unable to surrender totally to pleasure. I feel that I can't get enough, and that there is only a certain amount of time, so I feel hurried. I find that I am afraid of loving the man physically or in spirit. I can't see that they are there for me, even if they are. It's like I just know that if they are there for me, they won't be for long. I have opened myself to different relationships, but each time I proved that it is dangerous.

Biggest problem with sex .... Unable to surrender to the pleasure of it. I only had two orgasms with my husband (now my ex-husband) in ten years, and no one else since then. I still enjoy sex, but know it could be a lot better. I feel like a failure.

My Personal Lie .... I DON'T MATTER, I'M A FAILURE, I'M A NUISANCE, I'M NOT WANTED.

How my Personal Lie affects my sexuality .... I'll have sex for the man's sake—my feelings don't matter. In my marriage, my husband didn't support my sexuality—it didn't matter what I wanted. When I did ask, it caused too much unpleasantness, so after awhile I stopped asking. I can't orgasm, so I am a failure. I am not uninhibited enough, so I am a failure. I don't risk getting disapproval because I'm basically not wanted.

First memories of sexuality .... At age nine I was home alone. I had shorts on and noticed my genitals. I found out that it felt good to touch them.

Church conditioning .... Sex is bad outside of marriage. Sex is unspiritual later in life. Sex is of the body and that is not good—it distracts one from reaching God.

Parental conditioning . . . . You'll get pregnant. Don't do it before marriage, or at least before you're engaged. A subject of unease—hidden and not talked about. I was told to watch out for being used. I don't remember being told about sex. My parents never cuddled, touched, or kissed in front of me.

Most embarrassing sexual situation . . . . When I was about sixteen, I was parking with my boyfriend. We were kissing and he started to caress my genitals. He was either really fast, or I wasn't paying attention as I was too embarrassed, but before I knew it, he had put his finger in my vagina only to find a tampon there. He was horrified, and I was embarrassed, and felt dirty.

First sexual experience . . . . I was about eighteen. It was with my boyfriend of two years. He had gone to a university and I was at college. He had asked to make love for quite a while, but I always put him off. Finally I decided it would be OK, after my sister said it was all right to do it if you loved him. I travelled down to see him for the weekend. I had my period. I found that it felt average, not particularly enjoyable nor unpleasant. I was doing it for him—I felt that if I didn't, I'd lose him. I pretended to enjoy it, and did what I thought was required of me. I was a bit disappointed, and felt cold about it and powerless and naughty. I was uncomfortable with the other flatmates, and didn't want to be seen.

31. BRIAR

Conception description . . . . I was conceived on a boat off a small island. It was naughty and fun for my parents. They were with a lot of people, and they snuck away to have sex. I was conceived to replace my sister who died of cancer at two. I was born eighteen months after she died. The other girl was feminine and beautiful, and she died. My parents were afraid to really love me because I might die.

How my conception affects my sexuality . . . . I love making love on a boat, or doing it outside. When I think I might be caught is when I like to have sex. It makes it more exciting. Boats are very sexual and sensuous for me. Nothing else exists when I am out on a boat. I can become more intimate with my partner, because nothing else is out there. Sex on a boat is more naughty. People who are not supposed to get it together always do on boats. Alcohol is always involved. Alcohol was probably involved at my conception.

I acted like a boy to please my father. I wanted to be different from my sister who was feminine and died.

Birth description .... My birth was late, fast and easy.

How my birth affects my sexuality .... I feel that I am late for life. I was late getting interested in sex, and late masturbating. When my friends were having babies, I finally got married at twenty-three.

Sex for me is easy with women. It takes a long time for me to have an orgasm. I felt guilty when I was married. I didn't know how to please my husband, or how to be pleased by him. I just gave up and decided not to have sex with him. I was a late bloomer in sex. I felt obliged to have sex with my husband because he was nice.

My Personal Lie is .... I HURT PEOPLE AND I AM GUILTY.

How my Personal Lie affects my sexuality .... I feel guilty for having life be so easy. What I communicate hurts people. I am afraid to have a relationship. I feel either I will be hurt, or I will hurt my partner.

My biggest problem with sex was .... I didn't like sex with a man, because I didn't feel alive. I wasn't stimulated by them.

My biggest problem with sex now is .... I don't just want casual sex, but I am also afraid of intimacy. Intimacy leads to demand. Relationships feel like death to me. I can't be myself in relationships. I go after unavailable women so I don't have to be intimate. I go after straight women, or women who are already in a relationship. I don't like to be affectionate. I want my partner to feel loved without being dependent on affection. I push people away so I won't hurt them.

Oedipal Period .... I always played with little boys. There were five boys who lived in front of us, and four boys who lived next door. We would play doctor and nurse, and I would wrap leaves around their "dingers". I had penis envy. We always touched each other clinically like we were doctors.

Masturbation .... I never really masturbated until I was thirty-four. This was after my first relationship with a woman.

Church conditioning .... I went to a church school, but don't remember any negative conditioning about sex. I didn't feel any guilt about sex.

Parental conditioning .... Dad joked about sex and mom laughed about it. I knew they loved each other. I knew they were affectionate, but they sometimes tried to hide their feelings.

Embarrassing sexual experience .... I was in bed with this man I liked. I heard water running and looked down. He was peeing all over me and everything else. I was twenty-three.

32. ALISON

Birth description .... Late and long labor. I was three weeks late. My birth was a long, hard struggle. Maybe I was a dry birth.

How my birth affects my sexuality .... I create a lot of time issues around sex—it's never the right time, there isn't enough time to enjoy it, it's taking too long. Sex often seems like a struggle. It's hard to climax and I create being hurt by my partner, I don't like the missionary position because I feel crushed. There also seems to be an issue about lubrication. When sex is a struggle, that is often why. I feel irritated about being touched.

How my Personal Lie affects my sexuality .... I'm not wanted. It makes it hard to initiate sex—I'll interpret the smallest thing as rejection. My pattern has always been that sex is wonderful at the beginning of a relationship, and then about nine months into it, problems start.

I've certainly overcompensated sexually for not being wanted. I've had many different partners in many different circumstances, which has been a wonderful learning. I have the pattern that I leave relationships. It seems that I leave at the point when I have to admit that they truly want me.

My biggest problems with sex are .... There's never enough time for it. It's never more than just all right when we do make love. I am/am not pregnant.

Scheduling conflicts prove I am not wanted. If he really wanted me, there would be plenty of time for sex. Same with #2. If I was really wanted, sex would be wonderful. There's another payoff there. If sex was always wonderful, then I would want it more often, and if I had to initiate, then I'd be setting up many more chances to be rejected and unwanted. Not being pregnant just proves I'm unwanted as a mother! There's also that thought that if we had a child, the child would be #1 in Robert's eyes and I would be unwanted again!

33. ROBERT

How my conception affects my sexuality . . . . I enjoy sex. I easily express my emotions during sex. I am sexually attractive. I exude an air of danger, which is attractive to the opposite sex. I attract wives who do not like sex. I have been promiscuous in the past. I often give mixed signals to members of the opposite sex. I have great sexual fantasies and dreams.

Birth description . . . . Heavily drugged; C-section; emergency; thought mother might die.

How my birth affects my sexuality . . . . I spent 38 years seeking a birth canal experience. There has often been trauma associated with sex.

I'm as cute as I can be in order to survive.

I have had a violent sexual partner.

I have had a sexual partner attack me with a knife.

I often feel pain around the tip of my penis after I have climaxed. (I am uncircumsized.)

I am loved and wanted by my sexual partners.

I like dangerous sex, and sex in dangerous places.

I like secret sex in public areas.

I have enjoyed group sex.

I have enjoyed multiple partners.

I sometimes go unconscious during or immediately after having sex.

I enjoy sex on marijuana, etc.

I don't bond easily.

My Personal Lie is . . . . I AM A KILLER.

How my Personal Lie affects my sexuality is . . . . I am afraid of the power of my sexuality. I tend to attract people inappropriately. I'm afraid I will "blow someone away" with my sexuality. All but one of my sexual partners have left me. I often feel guilty about my sexual attractions and thoughts. I am very conscious of sexuality.

The correlation between my Personal Lie and my biggest problem with sex is . . . . I am afraid my sexuality will hurt or kill someone.

"I am an innocent, holy child of God, and my sexuality brings light and life and sensuality to everyone and everything."

34. JOE

Birth description . . . . Breech and late. At the time of my birth, my mother had a lot of fear about my older brother, who was fighting in Okinawa during World War II. I did not want to be born. I was late, breech, and was not breathing at birth. The doctor thought I was dead or would die. I did not feel it was safe to be a male child in 1945. My father was glad I was a boy because he was a farmer and wanted me to work, in case my brother didn't come back.

How my birth affects my sexuality . . . . I was never sure I wanted to be a male. I dressed in my sister's clothes and was a very effeminate child. I always gravitated to creative interests rather than sports, etc.

I was awkward with girls when I tried to have sex. I liked girls and felt comfortable in their presence, but was always afraid I would make a mistake. I was terrified of getting my wife pregnant before we were married. I didn't want a mistake.

I have been a non-violent "peacenik" all my life, doing marches in the '60's, and getting involved in Montessori education in the 70's. Montessori is a peace movement in education. She was nominated twice for the Nobel Peace Prize.

My biggest problem with sex is . . . . I'm not assertive enough. I'm afraid I won't do it right or won't please my mate, so I never initiate. I don't want to make a mistake. Whenever I do initiate, my wife isn't interested. She is only interested when she initiates.

My sexual eternal law is . . . . "I am perfect and everything I do is perfect."

35. CHARLEEN

Birth description . . . . Forceps. It was long and hard and extremely painful to my mother. I was stuck in the canal and needed forceps to get out. My mother died two months after giving birth to my brother, who was stillborn.

How my birth affects my sexuality .... I think the end result of sex is pain for the woman. I think sex can also lead to death. I feel I have to beware of the sexual feelings I have toward men, because it can bring me pain or even death. I deny the pleasurable feelings of being turned on because it can cause me pain—pain follows pleasure.

I have created relationships where I've allowed myself to feel strong sexual feelings, and then intense emotional pain when the relationships have ended.

My Personal Lie is .... Either MY ALIVENESS HURTS PEOPLE or I'M GUILTY. I feel if I really let my sexual energy flow, I might hurt someone.

How my Personal Lie affects my sexuality .... I feel guilty when I have sexual feelings for men other than my husband. I feel guilty that I don't feel a lot of sexual feelings for my husband. I feel guilty that my body isn't attractive.

My biggest problem with sex is .... I'm afraid that if I lose weight and become more attractive, I won't let myself be really intimate. I feel my energy that I haven't really explored—it could be overwhelming to a man, and then the man would back off and be turned off.

My sexual eternal law is .... I am an innocent child of God and people feel safe and loved in my presence.

APPENDIX A:

Glossary

1. THE LOVING RELATIONSHIPS TRAINING (LRT) is a personal growth seminar dedicated to teaching you how to get, and supporting you in having, the highest quality relationships in all your interactions. There are more than 25,000 graduates of the LRT, which was created thirteen years ago by Sondra Ray. The LRT is one of the leaders in the field of personal growth seminars, and is offered in fifteen centers throughout the United States, Europe, Australia, and New Zealand.

Within a weekend format, the LRT provides you with the support, knowledge and technology needed to create and maintain successful relationships, starting with your relationship with yourself, the most important relationship of all. The participants explore relationship issues in all parts of their lives, including their relationships with money, career, family, sex spirituality, their bodies, and rejuvenation.

The Training is a journey through your mind. The decisions and thoughts you have made in the past about relationships deeply affect your results. You learn to become conscious of those decisions, and release the feelings associated with them. You are given tools to use for getting what you want. The Training includes extensive data, as well as many experiential processes which apply the knowledge to your own life situation.

At this time, the LRT trainers are Sondra Ray, Bob Mandel, Mallie Mandel, Fredric Lehrman, Rhonda Levand, Philip Tarlow, Mikela Tarlow, and Diana Roberts.

To find out how and where to take an LRT in your area, call 1-800-INTL-LRT or (203) 354-8509. Or write LRT International, P.O. Box 1465, Washington, CT 06793.

2. REBIRTHING is a breathing technique, the purpose of which is to heighten self-awareness, and stimulate the body's natural ability to purify itself. Discovered in 1975, it has been practiced by thousands of people throughout the world.

In a rebirthing session, you are guided by a professional rebirther to a fuller, freer breath. Your rebirther is your anchor who provides a safe environment, and a positive context for growth. As you breathe, you feel increased energy. As you relax, this energy dissolves stress and tension. Old memories leave your mind and body. Pleasure replaces fear.

At birth, when the umbilical cord is hastily cut, you form the pattern of holding your breath in order to hold in fears and anxieties. Rebirthing is a safe, easy and gentle way of feeling your feelings while, at the same time, locating and releasing unconscious sources of negativity.

Becoming aware of your birth script, you free yourself to reverse old decisions, and empower yourself to make new choices grounded in high self-esteem and spiritual certainty. Your excitement about life, rudely interrupted at birth, is renewed. Rebirthing is a way to rediscover your divine self and your innocence, as well as to remember your purpose for being here.

Rebirthing is not therapy or a substitute for therapy. Nor is it religious. Quite simply, rebirthing is a breathing process which deeply touches the mind, body and spirit. Call (800) INTL-LRT or (203) 354-8509 to find a rebirther in your area.

3. *A Course In Miracles*—"The Course does not aim at teaching the meaning of love, for that is beyond what can be taught. It does aim, however, at removing the blocks to the awareness of love's presence, which is your natural inheritance. The opposite of love is fear, but what is all encompassing can have no opposite."

The Course is summed up very simply in this way: "Nothing real can be threatened. Nothing unreal exists. Herein lies the peace of God." *A Course In Miracles* teaches atonement, which is at-one-ment with God. Many of us made a decision somewhere along the way that we were separate from God. This decision separates us from love, success, innocence, abundance, peace and happiness. *A Course In Miracles* is a 365-day course which brings you back to your divinity, and all the miracles that that offers. Many lessons from the Course are referred to in this book. For study groups in your area, contact The Foundation For Inner Peace, Box 635, Tiburon, CA. 94920. Telephone: (415) 435-2255.

4. LIGHTENING UP ON SEX WEEKEND SEMINAR is a workshop geared toward supporting people in reclaiming their innocence in their sexuality.

There is a lot of talking about sex throughout the weekend, which takes the charge off of it. The talk also allows people to discover that they are not alone if they have "trouble with sex". The emphasis of the weekend is on how conception, birth and early childhood decisions about sexuality affect our sex lives now. For information on this workshop, contact Rhonda Levand, 3770 Greenview Drive, Marietta, GA 30068. Or call (404) 977-3043 or LRT International, P.O. Box 1465, Washington, CT 06793, or call (800)-INTL-LRT.

5. AFFIRMATIONS are positive statements you immerse in your consciousness in order to produce a desired result. Affirmations will change your negative thoughts about aliveness, life, relationships, yourself, sex, money, your body, etc., to positive ones. In order to change your negative thoughts, after you have had them for twenty, thirty, forty, or fifty years, you have to spend time and energy thinking the new, positive, higher thoughts. We suggest that people write a response column when they are writing affirmations. That way, you will know when you have integrated the new thought completely, because you will no longer have a negative response to it.

Example of an Affirmation and a Response Column

I am good enough as a man.	My mother wanted a girl.
I am good enough as a man.	Women are more loving.
I am good enough as a man.	My mother made me wrong, and was disappointed.
I am good enough as a man.	Bullshit.
I am good enough as a man.	Maybe.
I am good enough as a man.	I guess so.
I am good enough as a man.	That's right!

Another way to immerse the new thoughts in your consciousness is to make a tape of your affirmations. The more they reach your subconscious mind, the more they become real and conscious. We need to edit our movie script with affirmations. We cut out, or edit, our negative thoughts by adding new, positive, loving ones. Once we integrate the new thoughts, we start getting the positive results in our lives that we always wanted.

APPENDIX B:

Self-Analysis Tools

The Mini-Birth Script and the Mind Map are two tools which can be used to discover your own decisions about your conception, womb period, birth and early childhood.

The Mini-Birth Script gives you a listing of thoughts and decisions people make at conception, in the womb, at birth, and as infants. Look the decisions over, highlighting or underlining any of them which you feel you made. To the right of each negative decision is the affirmation to correct it. Write out the appropriate affirmations, or make a tape recording of them.

When making a tape, say each affirmation in the first person twice, including your name. For example, "I, Rhonda, am wanted as a woman." Then, say the affirmation in the second person: "You Rhonda, are wanted as a woman." It is great to have a person of the opposite sex say the affirmations in the second person on your tape, if you can.

I use this mini script in consultations. It is a quick and easy way to get in touch with thoughts and decisions you have about your conception, womb period, birth and nurturing.

The Mind Map is more detailed. (See the example of Sam.) In the first column, you write a description of each event or situation: your conception, womb period, birth, and feeding and early childhood. Write any recollection you have, or anything your parents told you.

You can use the Mini-Birth Script to help you do the second column: the decisions you made about these events. The third column is for you to design your own personal affirmations in order to heal any negative decisions you made, and to unravel your personal "case".

Since you will have a lot of affirmations if you work with the Mini-Birth Script and the Mind Map, it is my suggestion that you make an affirmation tape as described earlier. You want to unravel any negative, unconscious thoughts you have. You want to make a new movie script for your life, one which is focused on ease, fun, pleasure, prosperity and sexual bliss.

Mini-Birth Script

DECISION	AFFIRMATION
Conception Thoughts	
I am unwanted.	I am wanted.
I am a burden.	I am a gift.
I am illegitimate.	I am legitimate.
I am unwanted as a woman.	I am wanted as a woman.
I am unwanted as a man.	I am wanted as a man.
I am wanted for the wrong reasons.	I am wanted for the right reasons.
I am a mistake.	I am correct and perfect.
Womb Thoughts	
I have to get out of here.	It's safe to stay and be intimate.
If I don't get out of here I will die.	The more I stay, the more alive I am.
Pain follows pleasure.	Pleasure follows pleasure.
I don't belong here.	I belong here.
I don't want to be here.	I want to be here.
I'm not supposed to be here.	I'm supposed to be here.
Birth Thoughts	
Life is a struggle.	Life is easy.
I can't make it.	I can make it.
I'm helpless.	I'm strong and powerful.
I hurt people.	I pleasure and benefit people I love.
Men hurt me.	Men pleasure me.
I can't trust people.	I can trust people.
I am not safe.	I am safe.
I can't let go.	It's safe to let go.
I am alone and separate.	I am connected to the ones I love.
Feeding Thoughts	
There is not enough.	There is enough.
(Food, money, sex, love.)	(Food, money, sex, love.)
I can't have what I want.	I can have what I want.

I have to wait for what I want.	I can have what I want right away.
I can't have what I want when I want it.	I can have what I want when I want it.

Other Personal Lies

I am a disappointment as a woman.	I am a surprisingly wonderful woman.
I am a disappointment as a man.	I am a wonderful surprise as a man.
I am not enough.	I am enough.
I am too much.	I am just enough.
I am a killer.	I enhance life.
I am dangerous.	I am safe.
I am evil.	I am divine.
I am nothing.	I am everything.
I am bad.	I am good.
I am a phony and a fake.	I am real and authentic.
I am wrong as a man.	I am right as a man.
I am wrong as a woman.	I am right as a woman.
I am not good enough.	I am good enough.
I am not good enough as a woman.	I am good enough as a woman.
I am not good enough as a man.	I am good enough as a man.
I am guilty.	I am innocent.
I am ugly.	I am beautiful.
I am stupid.	I am brilliant.
There is something wrong with me.	I am perfect as I am.

Mind Chart (Sam)

Event	*Decision*	*Affirmation*
CONCEPTION DESCRIPTION Illegitimate, sneaky sex. Mother hated sex. Dad liked having sex, he was horny. Dad got mom pregnant to keep mom.	I am unwanted. I am illegitimate. I am sneaky with sex. I am sleazy. People want me for sex. I am wanted for the wrong reasons. I am a disappointment.	I want, love and accept myself. I am wanted. I am legitimate. I am honest and direct sexually. I am trustworthy. I am wanted for the right reasons. I am an inspiration. People love and want me just the way I am.
WOMB DESCRIPTION When I was in the womb, dad wanted to marry mom because mom was pregnant. Mom wanted an abortion. Then mom decided she wanted to marry dad but dad did not want to marry mom.	I want women who do not want me. When the woman wants me after I go after her, I don't want her. The reasons she does not want me are my inadequacies.	I want women who want me. The woman I want wants me. Once I choose to be with the woman I want, it is the right choice.

Mind Chart (Sam)

Event	*Decision*	*Affirmation*
WOMB DESCRIPTION Grandpa interfered (mom's dad) and told them they had to get married. When dad decided to marry mom she didn't want to, but they did get married. After my parents married they felt stuck. They didn't want each other and they tried to get rid of Sam. After 6 months in womb, mother got very sick taking pills to abort him.	I am not good enough to be wanted. I overcompensate to prove I am good enough, then she wants me, then I don't want her. When they want me, they are not the one I want. I am not supposed to be here. I am a pawn. I am confused about being here. I am supposed to be somewhere else. What's the use? Something outside myself is trying to kill me. There is something wrong with me.	I know that I am wanted, perfect and good enough just the way I am, I don't need women to prove that. I am supposed to be here. I am clear I am supposed to be here. I choose to be here now. This is the only place to be. I have a purpose to be here. I am safe and immortal now. I am perfect just the way I am, wanted and complete.

Mind Chart (Sam)

Event	*Decision*	*Affirmation*
BIRTH DESCRIPTION Mom is drugged. Mom is snipped. Sam is jaundiced at birth. Put separate from mom.	I am unconscious especially in morning. I hurt my mother/women. I am guilty for hurting women. Something is wrong with me. I am separate.	I am alive and conscious. My life urges are stronger than my death urges. I pleasure and benefit women. I am innocent. I am perfect just as I am. I am connected.
EARLY CHILDHOOD Sam not breastfed. Fed on Schedule. Father leaves.	I can't have what I want. I can't have what I want when I want it. Men are not there for me.	I can have what I want. I can have what I want when I want it. Men are there for me.

Mind Chart (Do your own self analysis)

Event	*Decision*	*Affirmation*
CONCEPTION DESCRIPTION		
WOMB DESCRIPTION		

Mind Chart (Do your own self analysis)

Event	*Decision*	*Affirmation*
BIRTH DESCRIPTION		
EARLY CHILDHOOD		

RECOMMENDED READING

The Autobiography of A Yogi by Paramahansa Yogananda (Los Angeles, CA: Self Realization Fellowship, 1974).

A Course In Miracles (Tiburon, CA: Foundation for Inner Peace, 1975).

Healing Love Through The Tao—Cultivating Female Energy by Mantak Chin & Maneewan Chia (Huntington, NY: Healing Tao Books, 1986).

The Illustrated Delta of Venus by Anais Nin, photographs by Bob Carlos Clarke (New York, NY: Gallery Books, 1980).

Indian Love Paintings by Hilde Bach (New York, NY: Crescent Books, 1985).

Sex—Quotations from Bhagwan Shree Rajneesh, compiled & edited by Pat Lear (Woodland Hills, CA: Lear Enterprises, 1981).

Sexual Energy Ecstasy—A Guide To Ultimate Intimate Sexual Experience by David Ramsdale & Ellen Jo Dorfman (Playa Del Rey, CA: Peak Skill Publishing, 1985).

Sexuality Sexercises—A 30 Day Exercise Course For Lightening Up On Sex by Rhonda Levand (Washington, CT: LRT International, 1987).

Sexual Secrets by Nik Douglas & Penny Slinger (New York, NY: Destiny Books, 1979).

The Tao of Love—The Ancient Chinese Way To Ecstasy by Jolan Chang (New York, NY: EP Dutton, 1977).

Books by Bob Mandel

Birth and Relationships, co-authored with Sondra Ray (Berkeley, CA: Celestial Arts, 1987).

Heart Over Heels (1989).

Money Mantras (Washington, CT: Open Heart Productions).
Open Heart Therapy (Berkeley, CA: Celestial Arts, 1984).
Two Hearts Are Better Than One (1986).

Books by Sondra Ray

Celebration of Breath (Berkeley, CA: Celestial Arts, 1983).
Drinking The Divine (1984).
How To Be Chic and Fabulous and Live Forever (1980).
Ideal Birth (1985).
I Deserve Love (1976).
Inner Communion (1990).
Loving Relationships (1980).
The Only Diet There Is (1981).
Pure Joy (1988).
Rebirthing In The New Age, co-authored with Leonard Orr (1983).

RECOMMENDED LISTENING

Tapes by Bob & Mallie Mandel, Open Heart Productions

"Amazing You"

"God Provides"

"Having It All"

"Money Mantras"

"Peace With Passion"

Tapes by Yves & Vince Betar, LRT International

"Being Here"

"Forgiveness"

Tape by Rhonda Levand & Jeffrey Baker

"Sexual Innocence"

Tapes by Sondra Ray, Life Unlimited

"Your Ideal Loving Relationship With Your Body & Weight"

"Your Ideal Loving Relationship With Money"

"Your Ideal Loving Relationship With Sex"

You can get all these tapes from the LRT International, P.O. Box 1465, Washington, CT 06793. Telephone: (800) INTL-LRT.